DOCUMENTING PATIENT CARE RESPONSIBLY

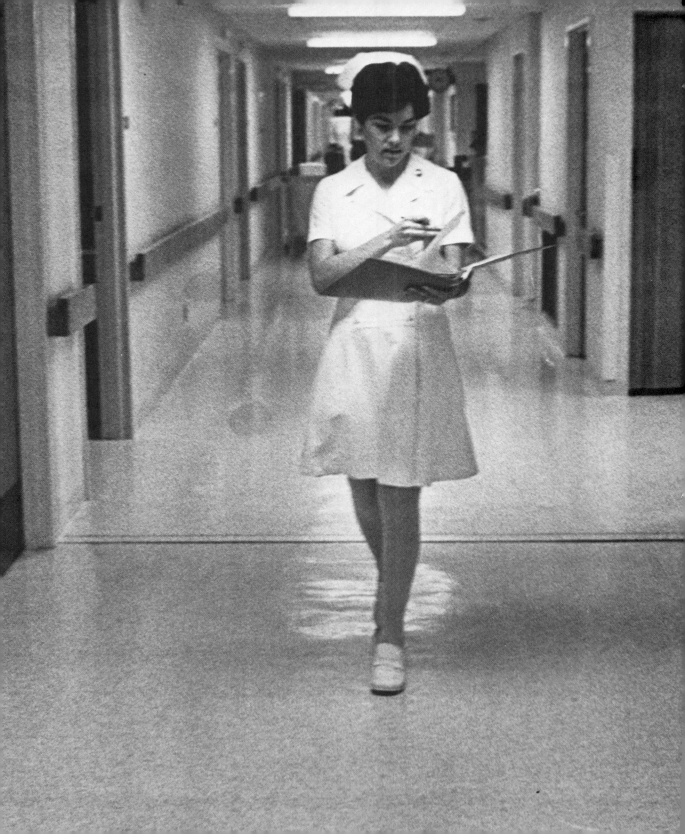

Documenting Patient Care Responsibly

NURSING 78 BOOKS
INTERMED COMMUNICATIONS, INC.
HORSHAM, PENNSYLVANIA

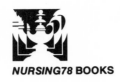

NURSING78 BOOKS

PUBLISHER: Eugene W. Jackson
Editorial Director: Daniel L. Cheney
Clinical Director: Margaret Van Meter, RN
Graphics Director: John Isely
Business Manager: Tom Temple

NURSING78 SKILLBOOK SERIES
Editorial staff for this volume:
Book Editor: Jean Robinson
Clinical Editors: Mary Gyetvan, RN, BSEd, and Barbara McVan, RN
Marginalia Editor: Sanford Robinson
Copy Editors: Patricia Hamilton and Kathy Lorenc
Researcher and Indexer: Vonda Heller
Production Manager: Bernard Haas
Production Assistant: David C. Kosten
Designers: John Isely and Sandra Simms
Illustrators: Bill Baker, Robert Jackson, Andy Myer,
    Jim Storey, and Kay Storey
Artists: Elizabeth Clark, Diane Fox, and Owen Heinrich

The cooperation of the staff of Doylestown Hospital, Doylestown,
    Pennsylvania, is gratefully acknowledged.

Clinical consultants
Irene M. Lee, RN, BA, *Professional Nurse Consultant,*
    Daisey Associates, Cherry Hill, New Jersey
Ellen K. Vasey, RN, BSN, MPH, *Director, Professional Resource*
    Associates, Medicon, Inc., Pittsburgh, Pennsylvania

DOCUMENTING PATIENT CARE RESPONSIBLY
"Nursing Skillbook series"
Bibliography: p. 192.
Includes index.
1. Nursing records.
[DNLM: 1. Nursing records. WY100.5 D637]
RT50.D62   651.5   78-14232
ISBN 0-916730-10-7

CONTENTS

AUTHORS

Lynne Sandmeyer Bootay is a consultant in patient education and the nursing process for Professional Resource Associates, a division of Medicon, Inc., and works part-time as a special project nurse at Braddock General Hospital, Braddock, Pennsylvania. She received her BSN from Carlow College, Pittsburgh.

Priscilla A. Butts received her BSN from Dillard University, New Orleans, and her MSN from the University of Pennsylvania, Philadelphia. She is assistant director of nursing services, women and children's division, at Thomas Jefferson University Hospital, Philadelphia. Ms. Butts is a past contributor to the Nursing Skillbook series.

Avice Kerr is a medical consultant and writer, as well as a legal consultant on medical records. A graduate of the University of Southern California Medical Center, Los Angeles, Ms. Kerr received her BA from Long Beach State University, California. She is a member of the Orthopedic Nurses' Association, and a contributing editor to *Nursing78* magazine.

Barbara J. Kleeman, who contributed the material on fad diets in this Skillbook, is a nutrition consultant for Dairy Council, Inc., Southampton, Pennsylvania. She received her BS from Drexel University, Philadelphia, and her MS from Pennsylvania State University, University Park, Pennsylvania. Ms. Kleeman is a member of the American Dietetic Association and the Society of Nutrition Education.

Irene M. Lee, one of the advisors on this book, is a professional nurse consultant with Daisey Associates. A graduate of West Jersey Hospital School of Nursing, Mrs. Lee received her BA from Rutgers, The State University, New Brunswick, New Jersey.

Mary M. Reilly is senior program coordinator at the Colorado Foundation for Medical Care, Denver. She is a graduate of Pittsburgh Hospital School of Nursing and received her BSN from Duquesne University, Pittsburgh. Ms. Reilly is a member of the American Nurses' Association and the National Arthritis Foundation.

Lorne Elkin Rozovsky, who contributed the article on legal questions, is the legal counsel of the Nova Scotia Department of Health, and a member of the Faculty of Medicine of Dalhousie University in

Halifax. A graduate of the University of New Brunswick and the University of Toronto, Mr. Rozovsky has lectured widely in Canada, the United States, and Europe.

Angela M. Staab received her BSN and MSN from the University of Pittsburgh. She is a family nurse practitioner at St. Barnabas Health Center, Gibsonia, Pennsylvania and a member of the American Nurses' Association.

Ellen K. Vasey, one of the advisors on this book, is currently the director of Professional Resource Associates, a division of Medicon, Inc. A graduate of McKeesport Hospital School of Nursing, she received her BSN from Duquesne University, Pittsburgh, and her MPH from the University of Pittsburgh. Ms. Vasey is a member of the American Nurses' Association and the National League for Nursing.

FOREWORD

In years past, most nurses believed that a patient's care was one thing, and the *record* of that care was another. Still, not every nurse agreed with this even 50 years ago. At that time, one wrote: "Many nurses complain that the time spent in charting might be more profitably used in bedside care. Is this not failing to recognize that adequate record-keeping is part of bedside care?"

Today, of course, we can no longer choose between giving care and keeping records. We realize that the records we keep are not only part of our patient's care, they *are* the care. No one can really determine what's been done for a patient, how well it's been done, and what should be done in the future, until he examines the documentation.

The patient's record from the time he's admitted to the hospital to the time he's discharged may reveal quality care — or it may not. Right or wrong, good or bad, this record is the only handle we have on reality. The notion that "care is good because we say it is" is outmoded and unprofessional. What we must accept is this: Documentation means *done* and no documentation means *not done*.

Now I'm aware that a lot of you still have difficulty documenting patient care. You're not sure if what you write is meaningful. And you suspect much of it may just be busy work.

Well, now you can say good-bye to those uncertainties — because this Skillbook will help you. It puts documentation in its rightful place, as an essential part of the nursing process.

What exactly is the nursing process? You'll find it explained in this text. In fact, the very outline of this book corresponds to the nursing process, with sections on data collection, care planning, implementation, and evaluation.

To begin to evaluate the care your patients receive, you must first understand the nursing process and put it into practice. Which record-keeping system your hospital uses is always secondary to this. I truly believe that if you practice the nursing process, you'll document it in a way that's meaningful.

As you probably already know, because of my association with Dr. Lawrence Weed, I endorse the problem-oriented system. In my opinion it's the only one that not only corresponds to the nursing process, but allows meaningful audit and feedback. But I also know that the method of record-keeping used in many hospitals is the source-oriented type. While this makes sense administratively, it doesn't make sense medically. However, don't let the type of record-keeping system you use inhibit you from practicing and documenting your care according to the nursing process.

While I don't agree with everything the authors have said in this Skillbook, the book does speak to all of you. Without endorsing any one system as the "right" way to document patient care, the book seeks to improve your documentation by showing how charting relates to the nursing process. It contains many examples of good charting, as well as some examples of poor charting. It illustrates how care plans are written by giving you a case history to follow from assessment to discharge.

What are some of the other things that make this book so valuable? It offers practical advice on how to protect yourself legally, including the answers to questions you've probably wished you could ask a lawyer about your practice. It also contains a list of the most commonly confused abbreviations used in charting, as well as some helpful assessment aids. And for those of you involved in new forms design, it offers practical tips from the Skillbook Company's graphics department.

No matter how experienced your care — or what record-keeping system you use — this Skillbook will improve your documentation. Over 25 nurses knowledgeable about the subject have contributed to it. Won't you take the time to read it? I think that the time you invest will reap dividends.

— DONNA GANE MCNEILL, RN
Research Associate, Promis Laboratory
University of Vermont, Burlington, Vermont

HOW TO
MAKE THE MOST
OF THE
NURSING PROCESS

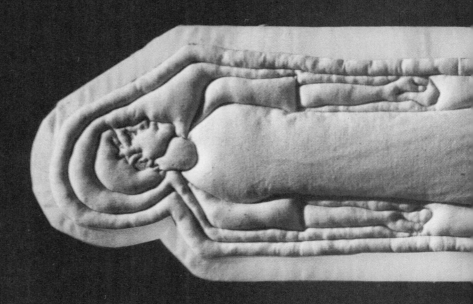

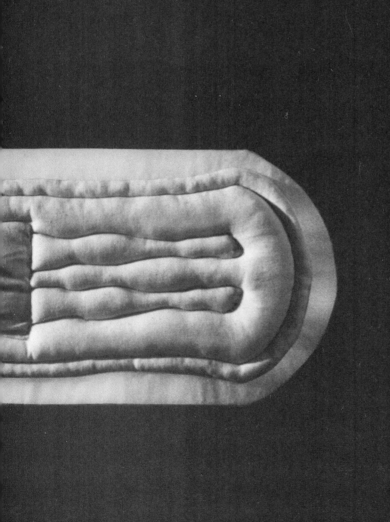

"Make patient assessment
an ongoing process in which you
continually review
the patient's problems and needs."

"Avoid standardizing
your patient's problems
according to his disease;
think of him as an individual."

"The problem-oriented system
of record-keeping
focuses on the problems
of the patient,
rather than
the source of information."

"In the source-oriented system,
each professional group —
or source — keeps its data
separate from the other
professional groups or sources."

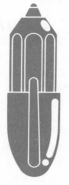

UNDERSTANDING THE NURSING PROCESS
Why it helps

BY PRISCILLA A. BUTTS, RN, MSN

TRY A LITTLE EXPERIMENT tomorrow. Ask three or four nurses in your unit what the term "nursing process" means to them. You may get some surprising answers, though most will be at least partially correct.

One nurse may say it has something to do with quality assurance; another may say it's a scientific method. Still another will say it's all about data collection and nursing assessment.

A set of building components

What *is* the nursing process? Do you understand it well enough to put it into words? Can you see how it encompasses *all* of the above answers — and makes them fit together? If you still think of it as just a theory, this chapter will help you change your mind about it. You'll see the nursing process as a set of building components, which — put together properly — will form a structure called Quality Care.

That, of course, implies you'll have problems to solve. Providing individualized quality care for each patient *always* involves problems. And that's where the scientific method of problem-solving enters into the picture: It's your blueprint to

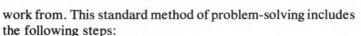

work from. This standard method of problem-solving includes the following steps:
- observing and recognizing the problem
- defining the problem
- arriving at possible solutions to the problem
- putting those solutions to work
- determining if those solutions have been successful.

Knowing where to begin
Now, let's take that blueprint and apply it to your job as a nurse, which is to build a structure of individualized quality care. Imagine each step linked to one of the components in your nursing process.

For example, in the first step, you must observe and recognize the problem. As a nurse, you do this when you collect and document data for your patient's initial assessment, as described in Chapters 3, 4, and 5.

In the next step, you define the problem you have to solve. This is where you make your nursing diagnosis, which will be discussed again in Chapter 6. *Your nursing diagnosis is not the same as the doctor's medical diagnosis*. You're not trying to identify the *cause* of the patient's medical problems. You're simply trying to identify *what each problem is,* so you can attempt to solve it.

Now, go on to the next step: arriving at possible solutions to the problem. This is where you figure out ways to solve each of the patient's problems — and decide on the best approach. After you do this, you write an individualized care plan that outlines the approach you've chosen for each problem. You will find an explanation of how to complete this step in Chapter 7.

Your next step is to put those solutions — or approaches — to work. This is where nursing implementation comes in. In other words, you take your goal-directed care plan and act on the specific instructions outlined in it. As you do this, you document what you've done for the patient and record his progress or lack of progress (see Chapters 9, 10, and 11).

The last step is this: determining if your solutions have been successful. In the nursing process, you and your peers do this when you evaluate what you've done for your patient and whether or not you've solved his problems. In other words, you take a close look at your initial assessment of the patient,

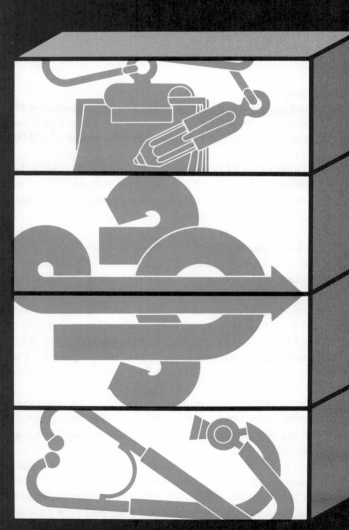

Blueprint for quality care

STEP 5: DETERMINING IF THOSE SOLUTIONS HAVE BEEN SUCCESSFUL. You and your peers evaluate what you've done for your patient and whether or not you've solved his problems.

STEP 4: PUTTING THOSE SOLUTIONS TO WORK. You implement your goal-directed care plan. As you do this, you document what you've done for the patient and record his progress or lack of progress.

STEP 3: ARRIVING AT POSSIBLE SOLUTIONS. You determine ways to solve each problem and decide on the best approach. Then, you write an individualized care plan.

STEP 2: DEFINING THE PATIENT'S PROBLEM. This is where you make your nursing diagnosis.

STEP 1: OBSERVING AND RECOGNIZING THE PROBLEM. You collect and document data for your patient's initial assessment.

your approach to his problems, and your implementation of his care plan. In this book, you'll find a detailed discussion of the evaluation component in Chapters 12 and 13.

Putting it all together
Now, put these problem-solving components together — in the order I've listed them — and you have the nursing process. Then remember I compared it to a set of building components that you use to build a structure called Quality Care. Keep that picture in your mind and you'll better understand your role as a professional. You'll know how to provide individualized quality care for your patients — by following a step-by-step process.

Avoiding the pitfalls
Let's consider some of the difficulties you'll encounter with this approach to nursing. Each component has its own pitfalls. And the sooner you know what they are, the better you'll be able to avoid them.

So I can illustrate what I mean, I'll describe your role in the nursing process more exactly. Your first responsibility, of course, is to collect enough significant data about your patient to make an accurate assessment.

Don't just be a collector
As you know, you collect data in three ways — by interviewing, observing, and inspecting. In the interview, you ask the patient or his family to describe the following: his reason for hospitalization; his personal health history, patterns, and habits; and his normal life-style. As you elicit this information, you strive to establish a therapeutic relationship with him. Winning the patient's cooperation is one of the purposes of the interview (see Chapter 3). Without it, you'll have difficulty caring for him.

You also collect data by using your senses — by observing and inspecting. *Like interviewing, this part of data-collecting must be an ongoing process that you implement each time you see the patient.*

Remember, however, to differentiate between these last two methods of data collection. Observing the patient and inspecting him are two different things. You observe by seeing, hearing, and smelling things about your patient's appear-

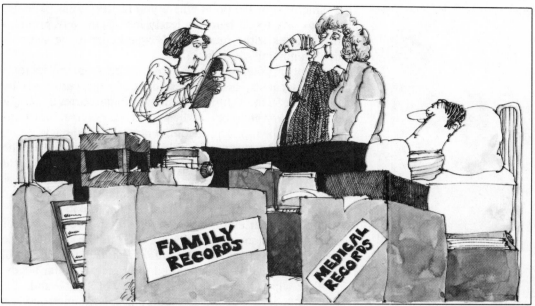

ance, movements, and responses. You inspect by using your sense of touch.

Now, let me describe the biggest blunder you can make during this phase of the nursing process. *It's forgetting why you're collecting the data.* To illustrate, I relate the obviously exaggerated story of Susie Collector, a nurse in a busy medical/surgical unit. She spent hours collecting data, by interviewing each patient, his family, and his friends. She consistently communicated with other health-team members, and requested old records on each patient whenever they were available.

Wasn't all this commendable? It might have been if Susie had come to any conclusions about the data she collected. But she was just interested in collecting it; she'd forgotten *what* she was supposed to do with it.

Moral: Know the real purpose for collecting data: to help you identify the patient's needs and plan his care. Collect data with that goal in mind and make sure all the information you gather is documented.

Making a nursing diagnosis

The next pitfall to avoid in the nursing process pertains to

Susie Collector
Susie's error lies in gathering information for its own sake. Collecting data is meaningful only if you use it to identify the patient's needs and plan his care.

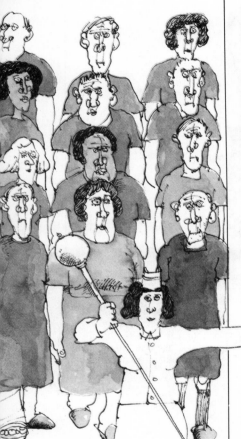

assessment — or the point where you identify your patient's problems. As I said before, clearly identifying any problem that interferes with your patient's well-being is the same as making a nursing diagnosis.

Remember, your nursing diagnosis differs from the doctor's medical diagnosis, because his identifies the *cause* of the patient's problem. A nursing diagnosis, made correctly, might identify a *symptom* as one of the patient's problems; for example, aphasia, hemiplegia, incontinence, and dysphagia.

In addition to this, you could correctly label one of the patient's *needs* as a problem. I think of cases when a patient needs extra help adjusting to disfiguring surgery, or when he needs teaching about prescribed medication.

But where can you go wrong identifying a patient's problems? You can attempt to standardize them too much. For example, a problem of incontinence can't be the same for two patients, because *both patients are individuals*. Each one will require a special care plan tailored to fit his particular needs. You'll see what I mean by this in my story of Sally Standard.

Sally Standard worked as a nurse in a large metropolitan hospital. She had special training in diabetic patient education

Sally Standard
Sally may be just a caricature, but the point she illustrates is a real one: NO patient's problem is exactly like another's. Always study each problem carefully. Then individualize your approach.

and taught many patients how to live with and manage their disease. One day Sally got a new patient, a young woman newly diagnosed as a diabetic. Sally immediately assumed that she was uninformed about her disease, and proceeded to implement her entire teaching plan for the self-administration of insulin.

What was wrong? Sally neglected to interview her new patient thoroughly before she implemented her plan. She just identified her need for patient teaching and assumed it was the same as any other new diabetic's. If she'd asked about the young woman's background and occupation, she'd have learned that her patient was a nurse in a diabetic clinic. She didn't need all the teaching Sally usually gave to new diabetics; she needed individualized help geared to her education level.

Moral: Never assume any patient's problem or need is exactly like another patient's, no matter how similar they seem. Study each problem carefully. Then individualize your approach to it in a way that will suit the patient's real needs.

Which approach is best?
Let's go to the planning phase of the nursing process — where you decide how to solve your patient's problems. Picking an approach can be difficult, especially if you have several alternatives.

First, you must list which problem deserves top priority, then explore ways to solve that. Compare the strengths and weaknesses of your alternative solutions, so you can eliminate ideas that seem impractical. For example, you may not have the staff or equipment you need to implement a specific plan. Or the patient may lack the resources necessary to continue your plan after he's discharged.

Many times the patient's learning level or personality rules out a specific approach. For example, you'd be unrealistic trying to teach a retarded patient how to administer his insulin. Or you'd be wrong insisting that a new mastectomy patient see a Reach-for-Recovery volunteer before she felt ready to.

So consider your alternatives carefully. *But don't fail to select one.* If you forget to make a decision, you'll be like the nurse in my next story: The Master Planner.

Rebecca Indecisive found it easy to identify each patient's problems, probably because she was so skilled at data collection. She asked all the right questions and documented meaningful information on each patient's initial assessment sheet. However, when she started working out solutions to each problem, she lost track of her purpose in doing so. She got so interested in writing ways to solve problems that she forgot to select one and put it on the care plan. As a result, each shift of nurses found their own way to take care of the patient's needs, and no one could tell which treatment was the most successful.

Moral: Always find more than one way to solve a patient's problem or take care of his needs. But make a definite decision which approach to use and indicate it on the patient's care plan.

Does your plan work?
Now you come to the action part of the nursing process: implementing your plan. Remember, implementation must stay goal-directed — with your expected outcome outlined in

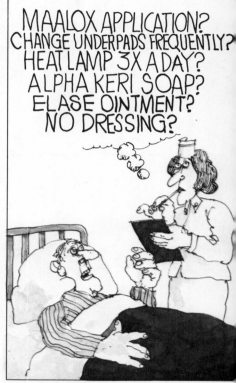

Rebecca Indecisive
Don't be like Rebecca and never pick a way to solve your patient's problems. Always make a choice and indicate it on the care plan.

advance. You must also set an approximate time in which to reach that goal, so you know when to try an alternative plan, if you must. Set a time limit that's realistic, flexible, and agreeable to the patient.

Never try to accomplish everything at once. And adjust your schedule, if your patient needs more time than you originally thought to make progress. For example, his physical condition may keep him from attaining some of the skills you'd like to teach him — or even from concentrating on them. I illustrate this in my next obviously exaggerated story about Zelda Speed.

Zelda Speed was a staff nurse in an Ob/Gyn unit, and she was exceptionally good at writing plans. Her problem lay in implementing them within an acceptable time span. One morning, Zelda entered the room of a 19-year-old patient who'd been delivered of a baby by emergency cesarean section the day before. Implementing her plan to teach the overwhelmed new mother infant care, she speedily demonstrated how to bathe the baby — and requested a return demonstration.

Moral: Don't try to implement your care plan at too fast a rate. Use common sense and make adjustments so your time schedule is agreeable to the patient.

Evaluating your approach

Ultimately, you must evaluate the ways you've chosen to solve your patient's problems. Have you met your goals? Evaluation, as a step in the nursing process, helps you determine the quality of your care and provides feedback on your initial assessment. Based on the results of the evaluation, you can reach any of these conclusions:

• The problem was correctly identified and the plan of action was effective.

• The problem was correctly identified, but your approach to it wasn't effective. You must implement one of your alternative approaches.

• The problem was incorrectly identified, thus making your plan of action ineffective.

• The problem was more complex than it appeared at first, so your plan of action was only partially effective. You need to repeat your plan for a longer period of time, or find a new approach to the problem.

Remember, however, that you must *document* how the

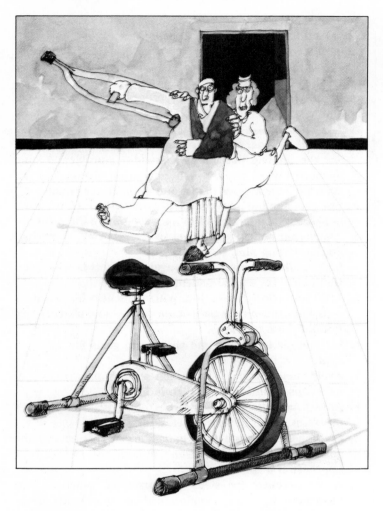

Zelda Speed
We'd never expect to see you doing this! In still another situation, in another unit, Zelda's zeal has led her astray: trying to implement her care plan at too fast a rate.

patient responds to your care — or you won't have anything to evaluate. I'd like to illustrate this point with the following story:

Three days after undergoing a hysterectomy, 50-year-old Mabel Whitney was still receiving meperidine hydrochloride (Demerol) 50 mg I.M. every 4 hours for pain. No mention of her response to the medication was made on her chart. When a nurse asked Mrs. Whitney to try an oral analgesic which was also ordered, Mrs. Whitney promptly agreed. "I thought an injection was the only thing I could have," she said. "No one ever asked me if I wanted anything else."

You'll learn more about the importance of documentation, as well as the differences in record-keeping systems, in the chapter that comes after this. For now, review what I've told you about your role in the nursing process by studying these ten reminders.

Remember these rules about the nursing process:
1. See the nursing process as a scientific, problem-solving method by which you assess the patient's problems, plan his care, implement your plans, and evaluate the results.
2. Use the nursing process as a systematic way to avoid haphazard planning, and to insure quality patient care.
3. Assess your patient's problems by interviewing, observing, and inspecting him.
4. Make patient assessment an ongoing process in which you continually review the patient's problems.
5. After you collect data on your patient, identify his problems — as both you and the patient see them — and plan his care to meet those problems.
6. Set realistic long-term and short-term goals for your patient.
7. Avoid standardizing your patient's problems according to his disease; think of him as an individual.
8. Always have alternate approaches for solving your patient's problems. Then be sure to select one.
9. Continually evaluate your patient's progress against the goals you've set for him. Don't be afraid to change your approach if it isn't working.
10. Never complete the steps of assessment, planning, implementation, and evaluation without thoroughly documenting what you've learned and done.

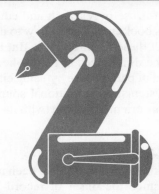

DOCUMENTING PATIENT CARE
How the systems work

BY ELLEN K. VASEY, RN, MPH

HOW DOES DOCUMENTATION FIT into the nursing process? Do you see it as something quite separate from the problem-solving method discussed in Chapter 1? You shouldn't, because it's an essential part of the process — the proof that your patient is receiving quality care.

A properly documented medical record should show everything done for the patient while cared for by health-team professionals. When the record's correctly documented, it:

• provides the data needed to plan the patient's care and insure continuity of that care.

• provides a way for health-team professionals to communicate with each other.

• furnishes written evidence of why the patient received the medical and nursing care he did; what response he had to that care; and what revisions were made in his care plan, if it proved ineffective.

• provides a way to review, study, and evaluate his care in preparation for an audit.

• provides a legal record that can be used to protect the patient, the hospital, or the health-team professionals who provide care.

• provides data for use in research and education.

Throughout this book, you'll learn how to document patient care so it meets all these requirements. But in this chapter, I want to explain the differences in record-keeping systems.

You can document patient care by using either of these two record-keeping systems: the traditional source-oriented system, or the problem-oriented system (with its numerous variations).

Source-oriented record-keeping

As you probably know, hospitals have been using the source-oriented system since the onset of record-keeping. In this system, each professional group — or source — keeps its data separate from the other professional groups or sources.

To illustrate, let's suppose you're seeking data on a patient, and your hospital uses the source-oriented record-keeping system. One part of the records will contain the doctor's orders, another will contain the laboratory data, and still another will contain your nursing data. To pull it together and get a complete health picture of your patient will require much time and effort.

The source-oriented record-keeping system has another time-consuming characteristic: It doesn't separate the patient's multiple problems. For example, a single narrative note in the record may include observations about several separate problems: one about the patient's urine output, as it relates to diuretic therapy; one discussing the condition of a cast on the left leg; and one reporting vomiting in relationship to a head injury.

Which order?

In each source's part of the records, you'll find a predetermined structure for filing data. For example, in the section you use, you'll have a definite order to the notes, although this order varies from hospital to hospital.

Let me explain what I mean by this. In some hospitals, the order of your notes may start with today's entry and work backward to the admission note. When this is the case, your initial assessment of the patient is filed at the very *end* of your record.

In other hospitals, your initial assessment of the patient gets filed at the beginning of your record. Then, subsequent entries about the patient fall in chronological order.

Unfortunately, professional groups — or sources — don't always agree on how they want the entries arranged. As a result, sometimes you may have to read a patient's record in two different "directions" — just to follow it.

Like other health-team professionals, you'll probably have difficulty reviewing the source-oriented record. Why? Because you lose precious time sorting out (1) the patient's problems, (2) the therapies ordered for those problems, and (3) his response to care.

Remember, you can improve your documentation — no matter what record-keeping system your hospital uses. For example, you can make your source-oriented records easier to review by writing them in the format we suggest in Chapter 10. Using that format, they include these five essential components: the initial assessment, the patient care plan, progress notes, flow sheets, and discharge summary.

Problem-oriented medical records

Many hospitals now use problem-oriented medical records (POMR). This system was developed by Dr. Lawrence L. Weed, a professor of medicine at the University of Vermont (see margin this page).

The POMR system differs from the source-oriented system in this important way: It focuses on the *problems* of the patient, instead of the *source* of information.

The problem-oriented record-keeping system helps health-team professionals in these three ways:
- by reducing their dependence on memory for important data necessary to the patient's care
- by preserving the logic of what they're doing
- by coordinating their efforts.

As an additional advantage, the POMR system's well-defined structure and order correspond with the nursing process. Ideally, this format should stay the same no matter which group of health-team professionals is using it. Included in the POMR format are these five components:
- data base, or initial assessment
- problem list
- initial plan
- progress notes
- discharge summary.

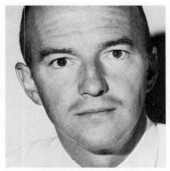

Looking ahead with Dr. Weed
Ever since 1958, Dr. Lawrence L. Weed has been working steadily to improve the way hospitals document patient care. The ideas he developed when he was in charge of Case Western Reserve's medical school have since become widely accepted throughout North America as the *problem-oriented* system of record-keeping.

According to its many advocates, Dr. Weed's system — if successfully implemented — will not only improve coordination among health teams, but also lead us closer to the ideal of comprehensive, individualized, personalized patient care.

Dr. Weed envisions a future in which every patient will have a "birth-to-death" problem list on record for use by any hospital. This list, available through a central computer bank, would provide health-care professionals with a patient's complete data base, anytime, anywhere.

Understanding the data base

Now let's examine this system, component by component, starting with the data base. As I said above, the guidelines you'll use to collect the initial data are predefined. They encompass these areas: the patient's chief complaint or reason for coming to the hospital; his personal and family history; his allergies, with a description of his usual reaction; his medication regimen at the time of admission; his physical assessment data, based on your observations and inspection; his mental and emotional status; and his life-style.

You must gather this data — and document it — as soon as possible after the patient's admission (see Chapters 3, 4, and 5). Then it's analyzed to identify his problems and begin to plan his care.

Understanding the problem list

As you learned in Chapter 1, problem identification is an essential part of the nursing process. No matter what record system you use, you should always identify your patient's active problems — although you may not list them with the source-oriented system. With the POMR system, you'll have a separate, well-defined problem list. It'll list not only the patient's *active* problems (chronic and acute), but his *past* problems, as well. And all health-team professionals contribute to it.

Later on in this book, you'll learn exactly how to identify your patient's problems by category, and how to contribute to his problem list using the POMR system. You'll also learn how to identify the patient's problem using the source-oriented system.

With either system, you identify problems only on the level you know they exist. A full explanation of how to do this appears in Chapter 6.

As soon as you number the patient's problems on the problem list, you can use these numbers to index your entire POMR record. To do this, make every entry on the patient's initial plan, progress notes, and discharge summary correspond to a specific number. When every entry has a number, no one can discuss more than one problem in a progress note. This gives the POMR system an advantage over the source-oriented system, because it's less confusing.

Understanding the initial plan

Once you've identified your patient's problems, you and other health-team professionals can begin an initial plan. This plan should include:

- the problem (and its corresponding number)
- goal or aim
- data collection plans, if additional data is necessary
- treatment plans
- patient education plans.

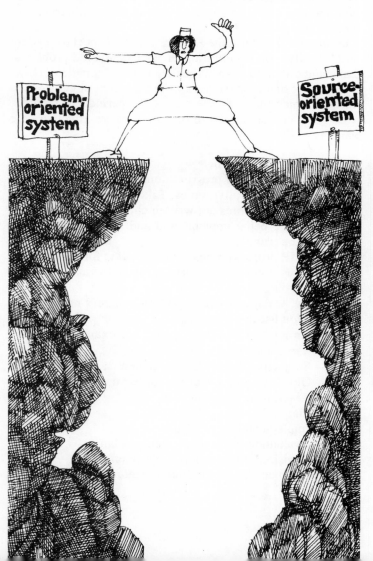

Bridging the gap

Recent innovations in hospital charting have made this a challenging period for nurses and other health-care professionals. As hospitals continue to adapt to new methods of record-keeping, you'll be faced with many practical problems to work out.

As you know, some hospitals have converted totally to the problem-oriented system; others are integrating it with source-oriented methods. Whichever situation you may be in, try to cope effectively with the demands of change. Your efforts to improve documentation are another way of showing your basic concern for the patient.

All health-team professionals should use these guidelines when they record entries on the initial plan. How the guidelines apply to their professional responsibilities varies. For example, you may gather additional data by interviewing, observing, and inspecting the patient. The doctor may gather additional data by ordering diagnostic studies. Similarly, you write treatment plans in the form of nursing orders. The doctor's treatment plans are specific medical orders.

In most hospitals, doctors' orders are not included on the initial plan, but are written on separate sheets. To conform to the problem-oriented record-keeping system, these orders must then be coded to correspond with the numbered problems on the problem list.

Do you routinely use the Kardex as a worksheet for patient care? Ideally, you should transfer your numbered problems, goals, and orders to it when the initial plan is complete. However, to save time, some nurses write care plans directly on the Kardex, which then become part of the permanent record.

To get a complete picture of how to write effective care plans, read Chapters 7 and 8.

Understanding progress notes

You'll use two types of progress notes in the POMR system: flow sheets and narrative notes. Like other POMR entries, narrative progress notes are written chronologically to show what plans are being implemented and how the patient responds to the plan.

The POMR progress notes have a specific format: They're called SOAP notes or, as they're used by many nurses, SOAPIER notes.

Basically, when you write a POMR progress note about a problem, you list the following:

• Problem number and description. For example, #1 Congestive heart failure.

• S — Subjective data (what the patient says he feels)
• O — Objective data (what you observe and inspect)
• A — Assessment (ongoing)
• P — Plan
• I — Implementation of plan
• E — Evaluation of the implemented plan
• R — Revision of the plan if it was ineffective.

If a problem needs specific attention more than once every 4 hours, record that you've completed this task on a flow sheet. Later summarize it on the narrative progress sheet. For example, if your care plan says that a postop patient must cough, turn, and deep-breathe every 2 hours, document your implementation of that order on the flow sheet, as soon as you've done it. Then, at the end of your shift, write a full summary in your progress notes under the letter I (Implementation). This will save time, and yet insure complete and accurate documentation.

Understanding the discharge summary
When the patient is ready for discharge, summarize what's been done for him on the POMR discharge summary. On this form, you take each problem on the patient's problem list and tell how that problem was resolved — or not resolved — when he was in the hospital. A SOAP note should be written for each active problem (see Chapter 11).

A discharge summary never explores a problem in depth, as progress notes and flow sheets do, but brings out only the highlights. In this way, it concludes the problem-oriented record and serves as:
- a reference for future problems (new or recurring)
- a way to transfer information to other hospitals and referral agencies
- a way to impart necessary health information to the patient.

Old ways die hard
As you can see, a great difference exists between source-oriented and problem-oriented systems. That's one reason why hospitals have trouble switching to the POMR system even if they want to. Many have adapted a compromise and use a combination of both record-keeping systems.

How are the record-keeping systems combined in this compromise? Basically, one or more professional health-team groups keeps its records separate from the others in a special section — the source-oriented way. However, within each section, they use these problem-oriented essentials:
- initial assessment (data base)
- problem identification
- initial plan
- progress notes
- discharge summary.

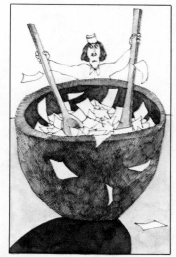

Weed salad
If your hospital's combining the source-oriented and problem-oriented systems, remember this: As designed by Dr. Weed, the problem-oriented system follows an ideally clear, logical sequence. Unfortunately, however, you'll seldom find the system in its pure form. Instead, you're more likely to encounter a "Weed salad" — in other words, a compromise, in which some elements of the problem-oriented system are grafted onto the source-oriented system. For example: You may number your patient's problems, but the rest of the health care team may not. Also, doctors may continue to chart separately, and may even use a different principle in organizing their patient progress notes.

Summing up

In this chapter you've learned how the source-oriented and problem-oriented record systems work, and how they're sometimes combined to fit the requirements (and realities) of some hospitals.

The rest of this book will teach you how to document patient care more responsibly, no matter what system (or combination of systems) your hospital uses. But before you go on to the next chapter, review these important points:

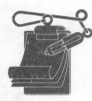

Remember these rules about documentation:

1. In the source-oriented system, each professional group — or source — keeps its data separate from the other professional groups or sources.
2. The source-oriented record-keeping system doesn't separate the patient's multiple problems.
3. The source-oriented system has a predetermined structure for filing data which varies from hospital to hospital.
4. The POMR system focuses on the *problems* of the patient, instead of the *source* of information.
5. Included in the POMR format are these five components:
   - data base, or initial assessment
   - problem list
   - initial plan
   - progress notes
   - discharge summary
6. Ideally, the POMR system's format should stay the same no matter which group of professionals is using it.
7. Number every entry on the POMR progress notes to correspond to the numbered problems on the problem list.
8. The POMR progress notes have a specific format called SOAP notes or, as they're used by many nurses, SOAPIER notes.
9. When a problem needs specific attention more than once every 4 hours, you'll record it on a POMR flow sheet.
10. Write a SOAP note for each active problem on the POMR discharge summary.

SKILLCHECK 1

1. Igor Mayakovsky, a 70-year-old retired seaman, has been admitted to your care with a diagnosed cancer of the lower lip. When you approach him, you find he's reluctant to speak to you. What do you do?
a) Identify the problem — he's embarrassed because of the sore on his lip.
b) Look further — maybe he doesn't understand English.
c) Respect his right to privacy — he's overwhelmed by his admission.
d) Ask that your assignment be changed — he's probably uncomfortable with you.

2. During your initial interview, you determine that Liza Dahlberg, a 64-year-old hairstylist admitted with urinary stress incontinence, is able to keep dry by voiding every 2 hours. Which of these beneficial actions would have the farthest reaching effects?
a) Offer the bedpan to her every 2 hours on your shift.
b) Record your nursing intervention on the nurses' notes.
c) Include the information on both the assessment sheet and the care plan.
d) Minimize this problem by restricting her fluid intake.

3. As team leader, you are initially undecided about the best way to help 48-year-old Ms. Koch safely and comfortably out of bed. She has a history of a fractured left hip and is now hospitalized for metastatic cancer which originated in the right breast. Whenever you ask her opinion, she replies "Whatever you think is best." What now?
a) Encourage your team members to develop a variety of approaches and report back to you.
b) Insist that Ms. Koch make a decision because only she knows what would work best.
c) Provide your team members with a range of possibilities and allow them the option of selection.
d) After you select what you think is probably the best approach from among the alternatives, instruct your team members to use it and report the results.

4. Mrs. Milton's problem has been identified on admission as safety concerns related to failing vision.

The nursing staff implemented the approaches listed on the care plan and documented them. You read in the progress notes that Mrs. Milton has fallen twice in the past 3 days by "tripping over objects she could not see." Which nursing reaction is justified?
a) Take extra precautions not written on Mrs. Milton's care plan.
b) Continue the same approaches for one more week.
c) Revise or add to the approaches on the care plan.
d) Change the problem on the care plan.

5. You're charting your nursing notes according to sequence and keeping them separate from other health professionals. Which record-keeping method are you using?
a) Source-oriented only.
b) Problem-oriented only.
c) Neither source- nor problem-oriented.
d) Weed method.

6. You document initial assessment information when a patient is admitted to your unit. Which record-keeping system are you using?
a) Source-oriented only.
b) Problem-oriented only.
c) Either source- or problem-oriented.
d) Neither source- nor problem-oriented.

7. Your documentation follows problem-oriented essentials and is kept separate from the doctor's. Which record-keeping method are you using?
a) Source-oriented only.
b) Problem-oriented only.
c) Either source- or problem-oriented.
d) Combination source- and problem-oriented.

8. You are reading a single entry in the nurse's narrative notes: It says, "Patient was bathed, fed, and assisted OOB for 20 minutes, which he tolerated well." Of which record-keeping method is this an example?
a) Source-oriented only.
b) Problem-oriented only.
c) Either source or problem-oriented.
d) Combination source- and problem-oriented.

(Answers on page 180)

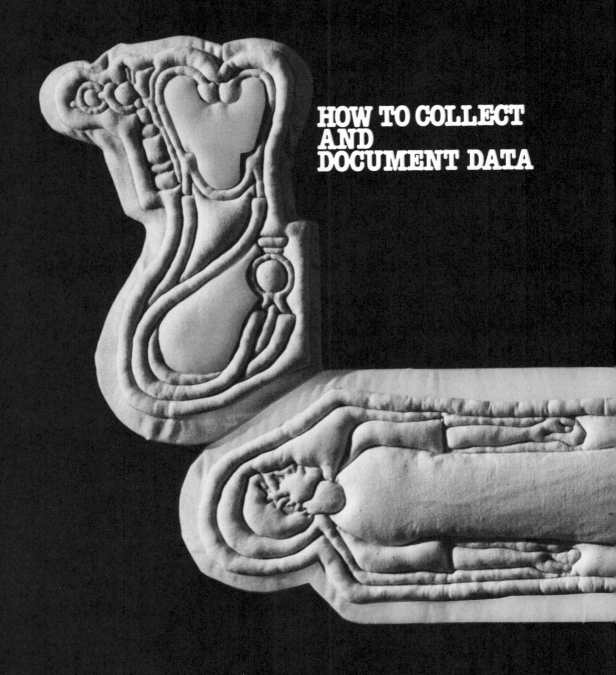

HOW TO COLLECT
AND
DOCUMENT DATA

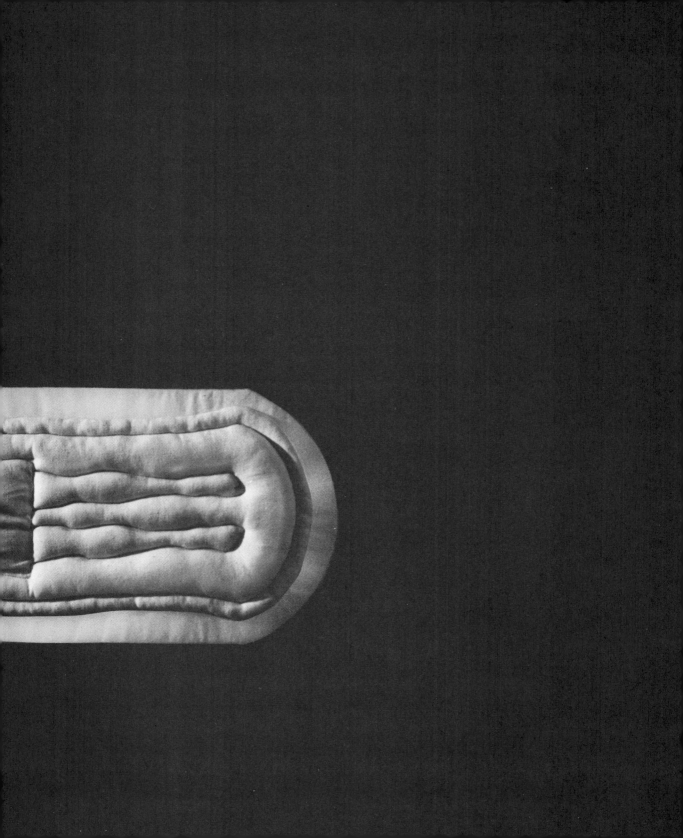

"Careful questioning
never robs the patient
of his dignity;
it seeks to maintain it."

"Know what you're looking for
when you observe
and inspect a patient.
Collect data
that relates to his problems."

"Your patient's personal habits
and health patterns
will affect his stay in the hospital,
so be sure
to record what they are."

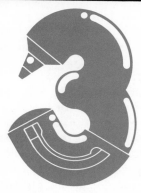

INTERVIEWING YOUR PATIENT
How to get the most from your questions

BY LYNNE SANDMEYER BOOTAY, RN, BSN

ROOM 221 SEEMS CHILLY to 82-year-old Anna O'Leary, as she sits with her legs dangling from the edge of the hospital bed. Only an hour has passed since she spoke to that snippy, young admission clerk. And now she's all alone, waiting for the nurse to return with the list of questions she said she had.

"Am I ever going to get out of here?" Mrs. O'Leary wonders, as she thinks of her home and the cat she left with a neighbor. Like so many other patients, Anna O'Leary has come to the hospital with built-in anxieties. Her discomfort since then has increased steadily.

Suppose you are the nurse assigned to interview and care for Mrs. O'Leary? Can you break through the wall of worries she's built around herself? Remember, the interview is the first step of the assessment process; how well you can communicate with the patient can determine how well you can write and implement her plan of care.

This chapter will help you improve your skills as an interviewer, no matter how much experience you've had. It'll teach you how to make interviewing the ongoing process it should be — and every encounter with the patient a meaningful one. You'll learn ways to enlist even the reluctant patient's

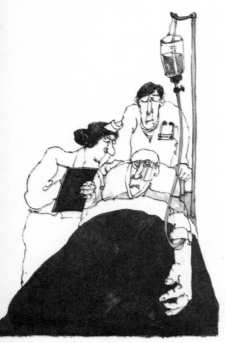

Wrong time, wrong place
Don't make this nurse's mistake.
Give your newly-arrived patient
time to adjust to his new
surroundings before you try to
interview him.

cooperation and make him an active participant in the interview. You'll make him realize how he benefits from the question-and-answer session, by explaining how it ultimately affects his care.

The interview: Where it fits in the nursing process

But before I get into the tips for better interviewing, let me review the interview's purpose. I want you to see it as a vital link in the nursing process — the first step in patient assessment. A successful interview will help you identify the patient's problems which, of course, is one of your major objectives. Once you identify his problems, you can make plans to assure him quality care. How skillfully you can tailor that care plan to fit your patient's needs depends on the amount and value of the information you get from the interview.

Unfortunately, some nurses still look on the patient interview — and its accompanying form — as written busy-work. But that's because they weren't taught to understand the nursing process as explained to you in Chapter 1. Your hospital's inservice department should start at the beginning and explain the nursing process thoroughly. Then you'll quickly understand everything else you need to know about proper documentation because it will all fall in place.

Understanding where the interview fits in the whole nursing process enhances your effectiveness as an interviewer. What's more, your patient will sense the motivation behind your questions and will respond more intently. Besides collecting the information you need about him, you'll be establishing a therapeutic relationship. These two objectives differentiate the nursing interview from that done by the hospital's admission clerk.

What affects your success

I've talked about your motivations for getting a good interview. Now let's look at the things that'll affect your success. These are your skills at:
 • explaining the purpose of the interview to the patient
 • selecting the right time (one that's agreeable to both you and the patient)
 • controlling the environment
 • putting the patient at ease

- implementing and improvising effective interviewing techniques
- concluding the interview in a way that'll make the patient an active, enthusiastic participant in his care plan.

Making a commitment

Just how do you explain the need for a personal interview? Remember, the patient's probably already answered the admissions clerk's questions. And he may have been interviewed by the nurse in his doctor's office prior to his admission. Help him to understand why *your* interview is different from these by explaining how it lays a foundation on which your care plans are built. This will show your concern for his welfare while he's hospitalized and show you're a person he can trust.

Once you've established your purpose for further questions — and the patient agrees to it — set up a time that's mutually agreeable. You're striving for a psychological commitment on his part. Keep in mind that being in a hospital tends to take away a person's sense of freedom. If you give him some choice of times for your interview — which is his right — he'll cooperate more, making the whole encounter more meaningful.

Don't make the same mistake that some nurses do when a new patient arrives. Don't rush into his room and announce that you're going to interview him. Give him a few minutes to get settled, then introduce yourself and ask how he's feeling. He may be upset about leaving his home and family, or he may be exhausted from a long drive to the hospital in heavy traffic. Possibly he's just had a whole set of X-rays taken, or has undergone some uncomfortable lab tests.

Suppose you sense your patient's too exhausted to answer questions — or tells you he is. Allow him his right to put it off for awhile — even if for only 15 or 20 minutes. If you must finish the interview before you go off duty, mention when *that* is, so he understands your time limits. Then set up an appointment for the interview, and return at the mutually agreed upon time.

Setting the environment

Gaining some control over the environment for your interview is your next step. Pay close attention to things like lighting, noise level, room temperature, odors, and the number of

What's in a name?

Your new patient is a woman around age 50. And you can't tell her marital status from the chart. Should you address her as Miss? Ms.? Mrs.? Or should you call her by her first name and risk her being offended? How patients like to be addressed varies. One person may feel uncomfortable if you begin a conversation on a first-name basis, yet another may be pleased that you've made a gesture to help her feel at home in the hospital.

Having difficulty deciding what to do? These tips should help:
- An elderly patient addressed by first name may feel that nurses look upon old people as children.
- A young patient may want to be called by his nickname.
- A PhD may prefer to be called "Doctor."

Remember, your personal sensitivity is your greatest asset in determining what to call your patients. The easiest way to learn is simply to ask.

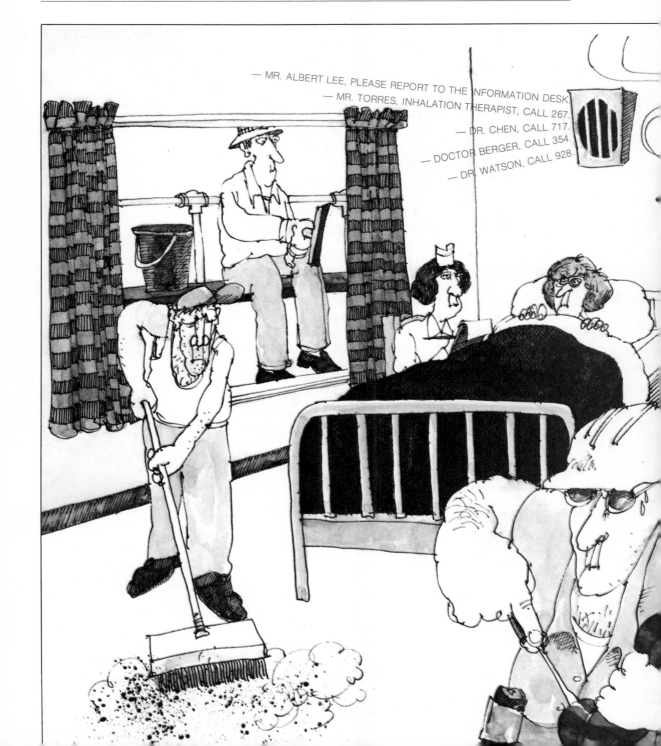

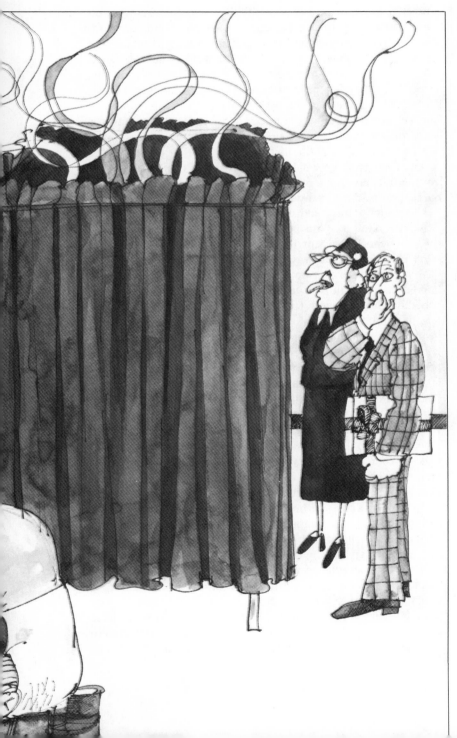

What's wrong with this picture?

Odors: Remove unpleasant odors before beginning the interview. For example, if there's a recently irrigated colostomy patient in the next bed, attend to him first. When you can't eliminate the source of the odor, move your patient to another room.

Noise: First, shut the door. Ask the patient's permission to turn off noisy appliances such as radios and TV. If the patient is unwilling to have a program interrupted, set up another appointment. If the source of the noise is beyond your control and the patient's, try to find a better location for the interview.

Lack of privacy. Provide a setting where the patient feels free to express his feelings. Remember that pulling a curtain between two beds provides only visual privacy.

Poor lighting. Keep the lighting moderate. Too high an intensity will cause eye fatigue, whereas a low level may induce drowsiness. Indirect lighting works best.

Uncomfortable temperature: Maintain room temperature between 65° and 72° F. (18.3° and 22.2° C.). Provide extra blankets or, when necessary, open a window.

Good timing

You'll always get the best results when you interview at the right time. In setting up an interview, these guidelines will help you:

• Always establish a time that's *mutually* convenient for you and your patient.

• Inform him how long the interview will take. No interview should exceed 45 minutes.

• Make sure he feels physically and emotionally well enough to participate. Don't attempt to interview a patient who's exhausted or in pain. If such symptoms begin to show during the interview, stop and continue later.

• Don't interview when either you or the patient are hungry.

• Don't begin an interview at the very end of your shift, when you may not be able to give your best.

• Always be on time when keeping an appointment with a patient.

people present. If any of these would prove distracting, do what you can to correct the situation. A distracting environment will make you and your patient uncomfortable, and neither one of you will give your full attention to the interview.

For example, suppose the patient's television set is blaring when you return for the interview. Ask if you can turn it down or off. Your patient probably won't mind the interruption if you've already mutually agreed on that particular time for your question-and-answer session.

However, let's say the distraction is another person in the room. Your problem will be more difficult. You'll want to give your patient complete privacy, but you know that drawing the curtain around his bed will offer him only visual privacy.

Use your common sense in this situation. If the other person is a close relative, your patient may want him to stay. First, find out who the visitor is, then ask your patient to tell you what he wants in the way of privacy.

When the other person is the patient's roommate, you can handle the situation several ways. For example, you can schedule the interview for a time when the roommate is on another floor for X-rays or sitting in the lounge area with visitors. Or you can ask an ambulatory roommate if he'd mind leaving you alone for a little while — just as he was given privacy when *he* was interviewed. If the roommate can't leave, perhaps you can take your patient to a more secluded place somewhere in the unit.

That all-important internal environment

Don't overlook the patient's *internal* environment — his feelings — when you're ready for his interview. How's he feeling mentally and physically? Is he in extreme pain? Is he worried about hospitalization costs? Does he have to void?

Perhaps he knows he has a terminal illness, and his readmission to the hospital means that his condition is deteriorating. That patient will probably be afraid of dying and won't be interested in answering questions he's been asked before.

But what can you do about the patient's internal environment? Probably a lot more than you think you can. First, of course, you can try to see if the patient's distressed — by pursuing verbal and nonverbal clues. One way to elicit these clues is to ask the patient what being in the hospital means to him. An anxious mother may tell you that it means her teenage

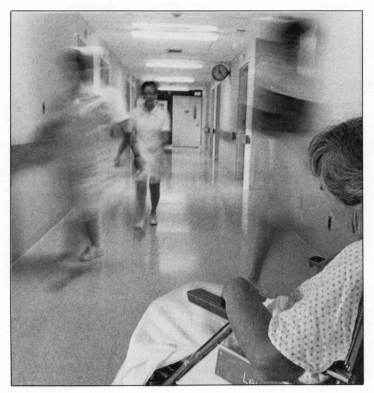

The elderly patient

During your interview, make your elderly patient feel more comfortable by learning about his expectations. For example, ask him "What does good health mean to *you*?" He may surprise you with his answer. To be able to get out of bed, sit in a chair, and watch TV may seem like a modest expectation. But an elderly patient deprived of these things may never feel healthy, no matter how well you care for him.

Remember, the elderly person's sense of time is different from yours. So when you question him, make an effort to slow down. If you don't, your behavior may communicate that you're in too much of a hurry to spend a few extra minutes with him.

Keep in mind that an adult doesn't become a child just because his memory is impaired or he has difficulty concentrating. Slow responses don't mean a slow intellect. What makes the aged person "different" is simply that he has lived longer. Try seeing him as a whole person, and many of your stereotypes about aging will disappear.

children won't have the supervision they need. A patient scheduled for disfiguring surgery may tell you that he'll lose his job.

Surely you can offer emotional support in cases like this. You may even be able to enlist the aid of the hospital's social service department for some problems. Or if the patient is worried unnecessarily about his impending surgery, you can teach and reassure him. Help the anxious patient who's being readmitted with a terminal illness by getting all the information you can from previous records. Don't burden him with questions he's already answered. You'll only sap his strength.

A sense of comfort

What you're striving for, as you concern yourself with the patient's internal environment, is making him comfortable. You want him to feel comfortable in the hospital setting and

TEN GUIDELINES
FOR BETTER INTERVIEWS

Your skill as an interviewer makes the
difference between a productive interview and
a nonproductive one. How do you ask
questions that provoke meaningful answers?
Which avenues lead to the most effective
results? Following these guidelines
will help make interviews better for both you
and your patients.

Q.   **A.**

Do you live alone?

No.

BETTER:
Tell me who you live with.

I live with my 70-year-old sister who is
bedridden.

Questions that stimulate explanations are more effective than questions easily answered by "yes" or "no."

*You don't feel faint when you get out of bed,
do you?*

Oh, no.

BETTER:
How do you feel when you get out of bed?

I feel like my head's spinning.

**Leading questions set up expectations. Anxious to cooperate, your patient may tell you what he
thinks you want to hear, regardless of the facts.**

Are your parents living or dead?

Living.

How old are your parents? How do they feel?

My mother's 59, and my father's
62, and both are still very active
and alert.

**When a question yields an incomplete or uninformative answer, rephrase it immediately to allow for a
fuller response.**

How's your hematuria?

Pardon me?

BETTER:
*When you pass water, do you notice
anything unusual?*

Sometimes in the morning, it looks reddish,
bloody.

**Whenever possible, use a common word or expression instead of medical terms. Clear and simple
language is one key to effective communication.**

*Do you think your husband's constant drinking
may have aggravated your hypertension?*

I really couldn't say.

BETTER:
*Can you think of any family problems that
might have aggravated your hypertension?*

Well, my husband's been under treatment for
some time now with his drinking problem, and
not making too much headway...

**Unless your own attitudes are nonjudgmental, your patient's responses will be inhibited. If a
question seems to imply a value judgment, think of a way to rephrase it.**

Q.   # A.

You know that not taking your insulin every day
can cause you to have your leg amputated.
Do you take your insulin every day?

Why yes, of course!

BETTER:
How often do you take your insulin?

At least three times a week, I think.

Implied threats and emotionally charged language produce fear, not answers.

Have you been admitted to the hospital before?

Yes, this is my third visit this year.

Your third visit?

Right, I was here in January and again in May.

You say you were here in January?

Yes, in January I had cholecystitis and then in May I came back because I had a cholecystectomy and now I have phlebitis.

Reflecting the patient's previous statement, or repeating what he has just said, will encourage him to volunteer more information. But be careful not to overwork this technique; it works best in small doses.

Why do you look so nervous, Mrs. White?

Oh, b-but I'm not!

BETTER:
You appear nervous, Mrs. White.   •

Do I? Well, I am a little worried that I may need an operation...

Direct "why" questions, especially about a patient's behavior, may create a defensive attitude. Just stating an observation lets the patient respond without feeling threatened. Give the patient a chance to confirm or correct your impression.

What time do you usually go to sleep at night?

It varies. Sometimes 10, or 11.

BETTER:
Do you have any special routine that helps you
fall asleep at night, so that we might be able
to help you carry this out while you're staying
with us?

Why yes. I always phone my daughter to let her know that everything's okay, usually just at 10. Would I be able to have a phone brought in?

Make sure your questions stress that the interview is designed to be *beneficial* to the patient. He should understand that his answers will help improve the quality of the care he receives.

Before we finish (looks at watch), Mrs. White,
is there something else you'd like to tell me?
Perhaps you have a question?

At the end of the interview, be sure to give the patient an opportunity to bring up additional information or to ask questions about what you've discussed.

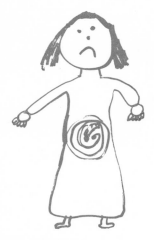

Draw me a picture
You're interviewing a sick child, and getting nowhere. His verbal skills just aren't adequate to describe what he's feeling. What do you do? Give the child crayons and paper, and you may find his answers to your questions highly eloquent. Ask the child to draw how he feels, or how he feels different from the way he usually feels. Especially revealing will be his body-image, the size of his drawing, and even the colors he chooses. Leave the paper and crayons beside the bed, and ask him to note any changes as they occur. In this way, even the least verbal child can give you a continuous record of his condition.

This technique can also be adopted for adults with speech impairments or language difficulties. Many patients unable to express themselves well verbally will find it reassuring to have a pencil and paper nearby as an aid to communication.

you want him to be comfortable with you as an interviewer. Many times this requires real ingenuity on your part and always it requires flexibility. But keep in mind that you have more control over the hospital environment than *he* does, and you can make various changes to suit his needs.

For example, let's get back to 82-year-old Mrs. O'Leary, who I mentioned at the beginning of this chapter. She was sitting with her legs dangling from the edge of her bed, which made her very uncomfortable. She also felt chilly because the hospital room was a lot cooler than she kept her house. She still rankled from her encounter with the admissions clerk and wondered if her nurse would treat her in the same offhand way.

How would you make a patient like Mrs. O'Leary comfortable for her interview? Well, you could start by helping her into bed. Then put a pillow behind her head and make sure she has a blanket. You could also bring her a cup of tea, or even offer to rub her back. Efforts like these impart a special feeling — that you see her as a person with needs and you're going to care for her.

In a sense, the patient is testing you at this point. He's wondering what kind of care you'll give him while he's in the hospital. So as you strive to make him comfortable during your first encounter, you're reassuring him and earning his trust.

Sometimes you can reinforce this feeling of personal concern by reaching out and touching him. To illustrate, let me tell you about a nurse I observed in a large outpatient clinic. Even though she couldn't take a distressed woman away from the crowded waiting room to interview her, she still made her feel set apart from the others — or special. How did she achieve this? By simply touching the woman's arm as she talked to her. The gentle gesture created comfort and made the interview more personal.

Of course, not everyone feels comfortable touching — or being touched. Use your own judgment and never intrude on a patient's space if he tenses up or withdraws from you. But try touching, even if you find it difficult at first. Your patient may need this to help him feel cared for.

See yourself as an interviewer
Now you're ready to ask questions. So pause and think seriously of yourself as a professional interviewer. Remind your-

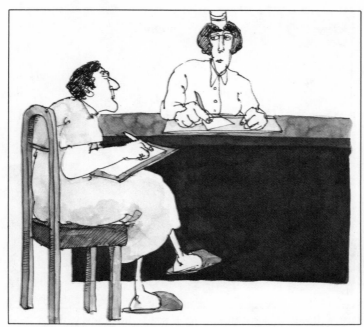

self why you need the information you'll gather to build your care plans.

Use the important techniques explained on pages 44 and 45. These techniques will help you get as much meaningful information as you can from every question. Getting meaningful information is what you're after, of course. If you can't relate it to any of the patient's problems, it's not that important to you. Never let an interview deteriorate into social chitchat. If you do, you'll have to come back for the information later.

A matter of privacy

Make sure the patient sees how your questions will benefit him, as explained in Interviewing Technique #9. Don't let him feel you're invading his privacy or seeking to change his life-style. The opposite is true — the interview is a way for him to preserve as much privacy and independence as possible in the hospital. The more you know about his personal habits, the more skillfully you can coordinate your care plans to his daily activities.

I'm thinking, for example, of a patient who always read his Bible before breakfast. In fact, he found it difficult to start the

Look who's assessing you!

You're not the only person gathering data when you first interview a patient. Your patient's gathering data on you and — from his impression of you — an impression of the whole health-care team. As you interview him, he's probably asking himself these questions:

What information does this nurse want?

What will she and the other people in the hospital do with it?

Does this nurse care about me as a person? Or is she just filling out another form?

Is she really listening to me? Can I confide in her?

Will these people respond quickly in a crisis? Do they seem competent?

What can you do to promote a favorable impression in your patient? First, ask yourself: Do I unintentionally send out negative messages? Do my voice, choice of words, posture, gestures, facial expressions contribute to a successful relationship with my patient? Or do I tend to avoid eye contact, to shift my weight, to adopt a cool, impersonal tone of voice, or to tap my pen impatiently?

By being aware of these or other hidden messages, you can overcome potential communication barriers between you and your patient.

Enlisting help

Are you overlooking a valuable member of your hospital staff? Someone who can help to implement your care plans, but who is seldom asked to make a contribution?

Consider the cleaning lady and how your patient relates to her. For example, your patient may feel more comfortable talking about his health problems to her than to you or a doctor. When she's in his room, he may tell her something that you should know, but unless you've kept your communication lines open with her, she may hesitate to approach you.

So when you see that the cleaning lady or some other nonprofessional staff member has good rapport with one of your patients, enlist her help. Make her feel that she, too, is an important part of the health team. And encourage her to let you know anything significant the patient tells her.

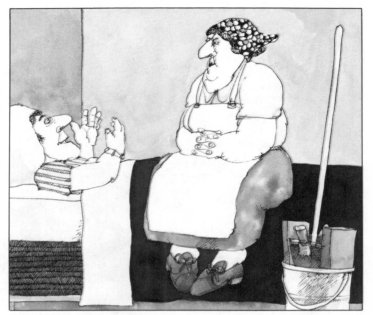

day without this routine. The nurse who knew this — and documented it — was able to assure him some privacy. Perhaps a patient of yours can't face the day without two cups of coffee. Careful questioning never robs the patient of his dignity; it seeks to *maintain* it.

Assure him that his answers will be kept confidential — that they'll be used only to help him. Then make sure you don't reveal facts about your patients in front of visitors, in crowded elevators, or around other patients. But remember that your patient has a right to keep certain information to himself. Never encourage him to reveal more about himself than he's comfortable revealing.

Curiously enough, some patients will tell you little and then confide at length in the cleaning lady. This is partly because the patient may feel more comfortable talking to the cleaning lady; she approaches him as a friend instead of as a professional. Too bad many nurses don't learn from this and, in addition, encourage her to share what helpful information she may have gathered.

What are the patient's coping mechanisms?

Keep in mind one of your objectives during the interview: to learn what the patient's coping mechanisms are. How would he deal with his problems if he were still at home? Will these ways interfere with the hospital routine? One elderly man I cared for was used to having his wife do almost everything for him. When we found this out, we could understand why he expected the nurses to act similarly.

On the other hand, the way a patient copes with a problem may help you write a care plan for him. A child, for example, can endure a lot if he has a favorite toy or security blanket with him.

Ask questions that will elicit this type of information, then make sure you relate it to the patient's problems. If you forget to do that, you won't find it very valuable.

Concluding the interview

Now you've come to the end of your interview with the patient. How do you conclude it? You don't just pick up your pen and paper and leave; a professional interview needs a proper conclusion. Instead, tell your patient that the time limit you've mutually agreed on is up and you've come to the end of your questions for that period. Then share what you feel the interview has accomplished, what you and he consider to be his needs, and what both of you plan to do about them.

For example, suppose the patient is going to have abdominal surgery the next morning and you now know that he's never had surgery of any kind. You've identified one of his needs — that he'll require extensive preop and postop teaching. Share this information with him and set up a time when you can return and care for this need. By doing this you reinforce what you've explained to him about the interview — that it helps you build a plan of care.

Sharing your findings with the patient in this way also gives him a chance to agree or disagree with them. And if he disagrees, he may give you further information that will help you even more.

So when you conclude your interview, do it properly so it'll be open-ended:
- Start identifying the patient's needs and problems.
- Begin formulating a care plan to meet those needs.
- Inform the patient about your plans.

Remember, make every encounter you have with a patient a purposeful one. A good interview must be an ongoing process,

Breaking the language barrier

Li Foong Ho, Maria Serrano, and Deiter Hauptmann share several things in common: Each was recently admitted to the hospital, none of them speak English, and all of them have to be interviewed.

Most patients who speak only a foreign language live or work with someone who can act as their interpreter. If such a person hasn't come with your patient to the hospital, he can probably be reached. But what do you do when no one the patient knows is available? Chances are, your staff includes people who speak a second language. In fact, the nursing services department probably keeps a record of them and of other people in the community who can serve in an emergency.

One way such resource people can help you is by developing a set of show cards with key ideas illustrated and labelled in all the major languages. Nursing Services can keep a few of these sets on hand for those times when you can't locate an interpreter.

When you interview, even with the help of a translator, always word your questions as simply as possible. Keep your questions basic enough to be transcribed into pictures, if necessary. Avoid using medical jargon. And remember, many popular and slang expressions contain double meanings which confuse even the most fluent interpreters.

if it's to result in individualized patient care based on effective care plans.

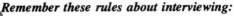

Remember these rules about interviewing:

1. **Know what an interview is for and how it fits into the nursing process. See yourself as an interviewer when you ask questions, not just a nurse doing busy work.**

2. **Explain the interview in a way that'll help the patient understand how it benefits him. Suggest that you establish a cooperative relationship.**

3. **Schedule the interview for a time convenient for both you and the patient.**

4. **Keep the environment as free from distractions as possible, and try to make the patient physically and emotionally comfortable.**

5. **Encourage the patient to communicate more expressively by asking open-ended questions, keeping related events in time sequence, and referring back to questions he's already answered. Never rush. Give him plenty of time to answer each question.**

6. **Use your common sense and sensitivity. Show your personal concern for the patient. Reach out and touch him.**

7. **Keep your questions centered on the patient's problems. Remember, you have to use the information you gather to write a care plan.**

8. **Don't insist the patient tell you more than he's comfortable telling you. Never imply that he won't receive adequate care from health-team members if he doesn't cooperate.**

9. **Look on interviewing as an ongoing process. Make every encounter with the patient a meaningful one.**

10. **Conclude your interview by identifying the patient's needs and share your plans about meeting those needs with him. Give him the opportunity to correct any misconceptions.**

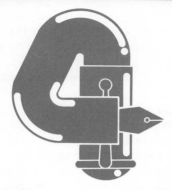

OBSERVING AND INSPECTING YOUR PATIENT
What to look for

BY ANGELA M. STAAB, MN, CRNP

YOU'RE A NURSE IN THE medical department of a large insurance company. And you're talking to 52-year-old executive Barton Freese, who was just brought in a few minutes earlier by an anxious co-worker. According to the co-worker, Mr. Freese doesn't look well and is having trouble breathing. Mr. Freese blames this on the big lunch he's just eaten. "I feel fine," he insists indignantly.

But you notice other signs. Rivulets of perspiration trace Mr. Freese's forehead. What's more, he's holding one shoulder stiffly, which suggests to you that he may be in pain. Mr. Freese could well be suffering an acute myocardial infarction, though he denies feeling any distress. "I have a lot of work to do," he tells you. "I must get back to my office."

Fortunately for Mr. Freese, you're skilled at making observations. Unlike an inexperienced nurse, you know what to look for even when a patient tells you nothing. If you didn't, you'd fall short in your final assessment of your patient's condition. The doctor would have more trouble accurately diagnosing. And you'd have trouble writing an effective care plan.

What makes one nurse more astute at observing and inspect-

Breaking it up
As you know, the traditional way of discussing the assessment procedure breaks it up into 4 categories: *observation, auscultation, palpation,* and *inspection.* Another way, closely related to the problem-oriented approach, is to divide assessment into observation and inspection only. Of course, all such distinctions are somewhat arbitrary: There's always going to be some overlapping. Usually, however, one element or the other predominates. In this book, we refer to any part of the assessment involving the use of touch as *inspection.*

ing than another? In this chapter, I'll tell you. And I'll explain how you can improve your skills so your findings relate to the patient's problems. These tips will help you write better care plans, thus ensuring each patient better care. You'll even find a list of ten of the most important tips at the end of this chapter.

Moving toward an assessment
You already know that before you can implement a care plan for a patient, you have to write that care plan. And before you can write a care plan, you have to collect the data to do it. Chapter 3 explained the first way you collect data about a patient, which was to interview him. This chapter explains the second and third way — observing and inspecting.

Let's start with the art of observing. To be good, this requires sharpened senses of hearing, seeing, and smelling. We define it this way: to see, sense, and gather information through careful attention. For example, you might observe that a patient is cyanotic, that his abdomen looks distended, or that his incision is draining. You might also notice that he wheezes, speaks with a hoarse voice, or smells bad.

How the patient communicates with you and others is also something you observe when you collect data. For example, does he express fear or anxiety? Does he speak angrily about his last stay in the hospital? Does he withdraw from conversation when you mention his upcoming surgery?

Anything you see, hear, or smell when you examine a patient is an observation. What's so special about this art? And how can any nurse fail to be skilled at it? First, she may be inexperienced or lack the knowledge she needs to seek out revealing clues to a patient's condition. Second, she may not do it systematically, and thus miss signs that would in some way be meaningful.

What's the third pitfall for a nurse making observations? *Not starting out with any goal in mind.* In other words, she makes no attempt to discover what the patient's problems are — even during a lengthy interview — so she doesn't know how to relate her observations to those problems. And if she can't use her observations to write an effective care plan, what's the sense of making them? She's forgotten that the success of the whole nursing process depends on her willingness and ability to tie every step together.

Start at the beginning

So imagine yourself with a patient. You're into the initial interview. And already you've begun to observe things about him that may or may not be meaningful. How can you tell what's important? Know what you're looking for. Read the doctor's admitting diagnosis. Then ask the patient why he's come to the hospital.

The two may not agree, you know. Occasionally, a doctor writes a diagnosis chosen to get his patient into the hospital faster. Though, of course, you'll suspect that when the patient tells you he's in the hospital for something quite different. Or the patient may tell you he's in "for tests," when the admitting diagnosis suggests cancer. Always double-check one reason against the other when you interview the patient, so you'll know what signs and symptoms to look for.

Let's consider that patient who says he's in "for tests." You obviously aren't going to tell him what his admitting diagnosis suggested. But you'll have to observe more than lab reports, so you'd better ask him to describe his problems to you. If he says he has severe back pain, then you begin by making observations about that back pain. You eventually write a care plan for that problem based on what you've learned from the initial assessment.

Before you make any further observations, always ask *how long* a patient's had a particular problem. That'll help you know what to look for next. Suppose, for example, that a patient comes in with moderate abnormal vaginal bleeding. Has she been bleeding for 2 hours or 2 months? If she's been bleeding for 2 months, you'd better look for signs of anemia. You may also need to write a special care plan to insure her safety in case she suffers dizziness.

Observe systematically

Use a systematic approach when you observe a patient. Then you're less likely to forget something. Start from his head and work your way down, as shown on page 188, unless common sense tells you to do otherwise.

First, get a general impression of the patient's appearance in a body area, then zero in on particulars. For example, check out his body symmetry before you make an observation about his limp.

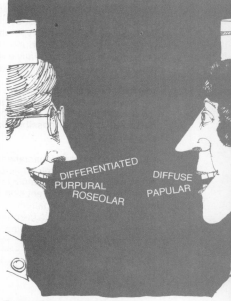

DIFFERENTIATED
PURPURAL
ROSEOLAR
DIFFUSE
PAPULAR

Expanding your vocabulary
Psychologists tell us that our vocabulary largely determines what we see. The more precisely we use words, the clearer our mental pictures become. As a nurse, the more accurate the words you use, the more likely you are to observe and record significant visual clues about your patient's condition.

Try this simple exercise to develop your vocabulary: Think of all the words you know to describe different skin conditions, such as *diffuse, roseolar, purpural, differentiated, papular,* etc. You can do this with a partner. Take turns naming descriptive adjectives for skin conditions until one of you is unable to continue. In this way, by repeating the exercise with words related to size, shape, spatial relations, movement, speed, gradation, and quantity, you can sharpen your verbal and visual skills. All it takes is just a few minutes a day.

SKIN PICTURES

Some hospitals now use this special data base chart to illustrate a new patient's skin condition. Just by writing the appropriate initial on the diagram, you indicate the type and position of any lesion. Then you can write a more detailed description in the accompanying assessment form. Such a chart can be especially useful in geriatric facilities, where patients commonly have skin abnormalities.

Risk factors in skin breakdown

Your assessment of your patient's skin condition should not stop here. Even if he doesn't have a skin condition now, he may be a candidate for skin breakdown. Watch for possible skin breakdown if your patient has any of the following:
- advanced age
- malnourishment or emaciation
- loss of excretory, skeletal, neuromuscular, and/or vascular control
- redness, swelling, or pain over a pressure point

   Start measures to prevent skin breakdown early and make sure to document them on the patient's care plan.

   If you wish, you may use the chart on the opposite page. It's been designed to reproduce on office copiers.

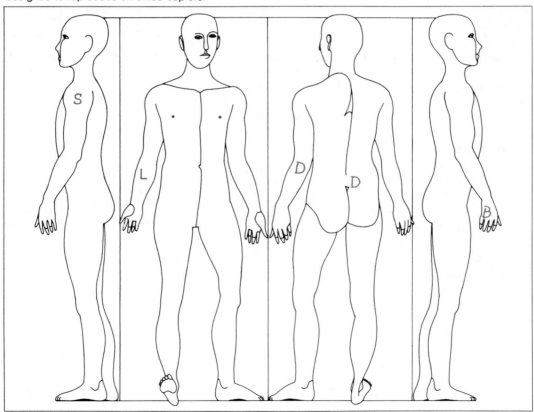

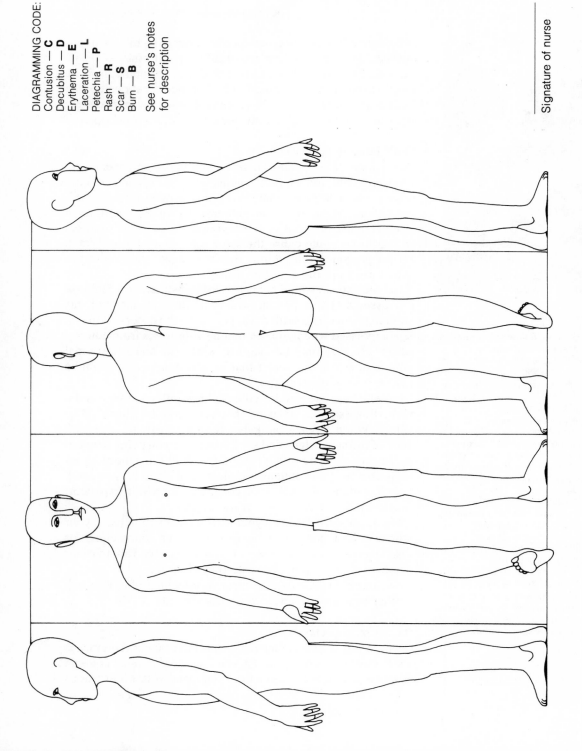

Signature of nurse

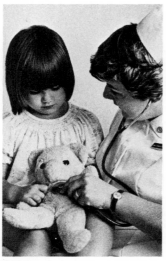

At ease
To make your patient more
comfortable during the
inspection, follow these rules:
• A small child may have a
stuffed toy with him. Put him at
ease by "examining" his toy first. If
the child's mother is with him, ask
her to hold him on her lap during
your examination.
• Always warm your hands and
all examining instruments before
touching the patient. Wash your
hands in warm water. (Remember,
some patients will be reassured to
see you practice personal
hygiene.)
• Always explain what you're
going to do while you're making
an examination, especially if it's
an unusual procedure.
• If any procedure is likely to
cause pain or discomfort, first
warn the patient. Then perform
this part of the examination last.
• Be prepared to spend more
time with an elderly patient. Avoid
seeming rushed; this will help him
relax and respond naturally.

Beware of the position in which he's lying, sitting, or standing. Are you sure he can move all four extremities? Is he slumped because he has an abnormality of the spine, or is he simply tired? If he's confined to bed, notice what position he finds comfortable. Don't miss signs that aren't immediately obvious in a reclining patient; for example, a foot drop.

Don't jump to conclusions
Never jump to a conclusion when you make an observation about a patient, even if that conclusion seems obvious to you. Always check it out against the other information you gather, as well as the information gathered by other health-team members. The best rule is to ask yourself what other diseases or conditions could cause the same signs in a patient. Watch out for preconceived notions that may make you see things differently from the way they really are.

Let me explain what I mean by that last statement. Suppose you assume that a patient will want to converse with his roommate once he's settled. Do you make the observation that he's depressed when you see that he withdraws from conversation? He may only be taciturn, which for him is a normal condition. If you document that he acts depressed, you'll be making a false observation.

Or let's suppose you let your feelings influence your judgment. For example, imagine that your grandmother died of cancer. When a sweet old lady is admitted to your unit with some of the same signs and symptoms, are you going to avoid seeing them? If you find it painful to ask her questions about her problems, you could miss collecting all the data you need. A similar situation arises when you feel anger toward a patient; for example, a drug abuser or an alcoholic.

What can you do to keep your feelings from influencing your judgment? Get them out in the open. Examine your feelings for what they are, and try to see them objectively. Talk to other members of the staff about it; they may have had similar problems. If you still can't control your feelings after this, ask another nurse to complete your assessment.

The art of inspection
The third way to collect data is to inspect the patient. This means you'll view him closely, using your *sense of touch*. You can inspect a patient at the same time you make your observations

and complete your interview. The important thing to remember is that you *touch* the area you want to inspect. *In my opinion, you haven't made a proper inspection without that.*

For example, you'll rub your hand over a rash if you see one on your patient. You'll feel if it's dry, wet, scaly, or crusty. You'll estimate how deep it is, and whether or not it contains fluid. You can also tell if it hurts the patient, and possibly if it itches him. In other words, you'll get a complete picture of that rash on which to build a plan of care.

Of course, the patient's skin isn't the only area you'll inspect (see pages 54 and 55). You'll use touch to palpate his abdomen. You'll test the strength of his grip in both extremities, and you'll feel his pulses. You'll use a tongue depressor to look inside the patient's mouth, and a stethoscope to listen to his chest sounds. You'll feel his muscle tone, and you'll locate areas where he was experiencing pain.

Follow the same advice I gave you about observing the patient — do your inspection systematically. And know what you're looking for before you begin, so you can relate it to the patient's problems. Don't let preconceived notions about a disease or condition keep you from making a thorough inspection. Don't let your feelings about a particular patient interfere with this part of your assessment.

When touching's a problem
I know touching can be a difficult problem for some people. That's why some nurses try to do inspections without it. Instead, they rely on their observations as much as they can and trust the patient to supply them with needed data.

Don't let touching be a problem for you. Your inspection isn't complete without it. And without a complete inspection as part of your initial assessment, you won't be able to write an effective plan of care.

Follow your hunches
I'd like to mention one more thing to remember before I finish this chapter: Follow your hunches. Your intuition is your sixth sense, according to some people, and it's worth paying attention to. For example, suppose a patient's signs and symptoms point in one direction, but your intuition points in another. Check out that creative hunch, but don't act on it till you get all the facts.

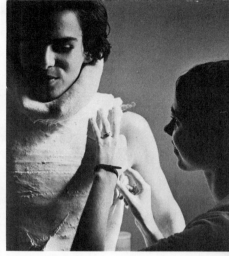

Tips on touching
Touching's an important part of nursing care, not only as a vital aid to assessment, but also as a form of communication. When understood as a caring, supportive gesture, touch can help break down communication barriers between you and your patient.

Here are some points to remember about touching:
• The way people tolerate and interpret touch varies with their previous experience, cultural background, and social maturity. Using touch effectively requires discretion and sensitivity.
• Unless your verbal and nonverbal behavior are in harmony, your sincerity will be open to question. An angry tone of voice coupled with a gesture intended to convey comfort and support would be meaningless.
• Just as you'll try to sense each patient's attitude toward touching, try to be aware of your own feelings about it. Use touching only when you and your patient are comfortable in doing so.

Putting it all together

Now you've completed your initial observation and inspection of your patient. You're ready to make it count for something. And it will, if you've related your findings to the patient's problems. If you have, you can use that data to build an effective plan of care. What's more, you'll have an accurate and complete baseline on that patient to compare with future observations and inspections.

Remember these rules about observing and inspecting:

1. **Know what you're looking for when you observe and inspect a patient. Collect data that relates to his problems.**
2. **Observe and inspect systematically. Get a general impression of the patient's condition and then zero in on particulars.**
3. **Never jump to conclusions about your findings. Ask yourself "What other disease or condition could cause the same signs and symptoms?"**
4. **Don't let your preconceived ideas about people or their problems influence your judgment or keep you from doing a complete assessment.**
5. **Examine your own feelings about a patient and his problems so you can recognize any difficulties you'll have making a thorough assessment.**
6. **Don't neglect the sense of touch when you inspect a patient. You can't make a proper inspection without it.**
7. **Follow up on creative hunches when you have them, even if they seem farfetched. However, never act on those hunches till you get all the facts.**
8. **Make observing and inspecting an ongoing process. Use your initial finding only to establish a baseline.**
9. **Identify the patient's problem or problems first; then look for additional data that'll help you write a care plan.**
10. **Understand why observing and inspecting is so important. See it as a vital link in the entire nursing process.**

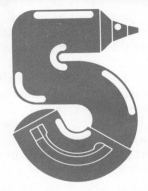

DOCUMENTING
THE INITIAL ASSESSMENT
What to write

BY MARY M. REILLY, RN, BSN

IMAGINE YOURSELF WRITING OUT an incident report. Why? Because an 85-year-old patient, who was just admitted to your unit yesterday, fell out of bed and fractured his hip. The accident occurred because he had to void during the night and couldn't climb over the upraised bed rails. It could have been avoided if the admitting nurse had documented that he normally got up at least once a night when she made her initial assessment.

The reasons for good documentation

Interviewing, observing, and inspecting aren't enough, you see. To have a complete assessment, you must write down the data you collect on the patient's medical record. If you don't, you're going to have problems — perhaps even more serious than the one described above.

The key purpose of a medical record is to give members of the health-care team a way to communicate with each other. If you don't enter all the information you gather into that record, you'll block that communication and interfere with the care the patient will receive.

So, besides providing a way to communicate, a properly

Focus on the problem

What do you do when a patient's condition is so acute that there's no time for a complete and detailed assessment?

Focus on the problem.

Center your interview on his condition and its history. Then limit your observation and inspection to those areas directly related to the immediate problem.

For example, suppose Paul Kowalski, a 43-year-old steelworker, has been admitted to your unit with acute dyspnea. You see that it's difficult for him to answer questions, so you try to phrase them so he can answer in just a few words.

Ask:

When did your attack start?
What brought it on?
Do you cough? How often? Do you bring up phlegm?
Are you in pain?

Now, because you know that pulmonary problems also have an immediate bearing on the circulatory system, you center your observation and inspection on both areas.

Observe:

Rate, rhythm, symmetry, depth, and effort of breathing
Appearance of sputum
Skin color
Condition of nailbeds
Edema

Inspect:

Breath sounds: i.e., rales, wheezes, etc.
Blood pressure
Temperature
Apical-radial pulse

Of course, if and when Mr. Kowalski's condition shows any improvement, you'll make sure to get the rest of the information needed to write a complete assessment.

written initial assessment serves as the following:

- a method to document initial baseline data
- a system which enables you to consistently identify each patient's problems
- a foundation on which you can build an effective care plan
- a way to prove — in court or to an audit committee — that you've given a patient quality care.

Why the old way wasn't the best way

Do you remember when you could condense all the data you gathered for your initial assessment in a brief write-up? In those days, you were finished observing and inspecting the patient when you took his vital signs and weighed him. You interviewed him with a few questions like these: "Why did you come to the hospital?" and "Do you have any allergies?" Then you wrote down the time he arrived in your unit, his room number, and a list of his belongings.

Obviously that approach wasn't an adequate one. We soon found out we couldn't develop proper patient care plans from it. We also discovered that many of the most significant facts about a patient came to light days after he was admitted. What's more, we had trouble communicating with other health-team members about each patient, because most of the information we'd collected remained in our heads. We had to find the nurse who could *tell* us what we wanted to know about a patient or do without the information if she was enjoying a day off.

As good nurses, we got increasingly uncomfortable with the situation. We knew we couldn't give each patient the care he deserved. And we suspected the patient knew it because nurse after nurse would ask him the same questions. Without proper documentation, we realized there was no consistency to patient care, because there were no defined procedures. So we decided to change things and examine exactly what we needed to know to plan a patient's care and what we needed to document.

The patient assessment guide you use today came as a result of all this. See the example on page 63. Though the format may vary from one hospital to another, all assessment guides should include the same key elements. These are:

- the patient's chief complaint or reason he came to the hospital and the duration of this problem

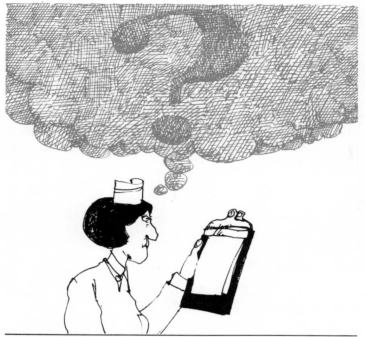

You've just begun your rounds on the 3-to-11 shift and you notice that one of your patients is breathing with difficulty. Quickly scanning his chart, you see no mention of his breath sounds. Did the nurse on the previous shift check them and find them clear, or did she not evaluate the patient's chest at all? How can you distinguish the absence of a problem from the lack of its assessment on a "negative chart?" You can't, which is why current practice has changed over to documenting not only care given, but also *all* pertinent observations, both negative and positive. To provide consistent high-quality nursing care, you need complete and consistent documentation.

- his personal and family health history
- his allergies, if any, with a description of his usual reaction
- his medication regimen at time of admission
- his physical assessment data, based on your observations and inspection
- his mental and emotional status
- his life-style habits.

In other words, you want to find out — in depth — who your patient is, where he came from, and how you can best help him adjust to his hospital stay and his eventual return to society.

Knowing what to write

Now let's consider how you'll document the information you've collected while interviewing, observing, and inspecting the patient. First, keep in mind that you can refer to this write-up by several different names. For example, you'll probably call it a nursing data base if your hospital uses the problem-oriented method of record-keeping. You'll call it a nursing history, or nursing admission note if your hospital uses the source-oriented method.

The name doesn't matter, as long as you remember that the purpose behind the documentation remains the same. It must fulfill the role I outlined for it at the beginning of this chapter.

As you know, Section I of most admission forms includes spaces to fill in general information like the following: the patient's vital signs, his height, weight, type of diet, and prosthesis, if any. It also includes an area to check if he's had lab work done before he came to your unit. It shows that you've oriented the patient to the hospital setting by demonstrating how to use the call light and intercom, and telling him what time meals are served.

SECTION I *

Mode __*Ambulatory*__   Date __3/1/78__   Time __1 30 p.m.__

T __99 6__   P __90__   R __18__   BP __140/100__

Ht __5'3"__   Wt __156__   Diet __1800 cal. ADA__

Bloodwork: Yes __✓__ No _____ Urinalysis: Yes __✓__ No _____

Prosthesis: Glasses __None__ Contact lenses __None__ Dentures __None__

Other __None__

General orientation to hospital environment by: __M. Adams, LPN__ __3/1/78__
                                                        Signature   Date
*Must be completed and signed by an RN or LPN on all admissions

If your hospital's policy states that an LPN or aide can fill in this section, delegate the responsibility to save your time for other demanding tasks. However, remember that the LPN or aide must sign it and you must review and sign the information she documents. If you have any doubt about the information, validate it at the patient's bedside.

When Section I is complete, you'll spend time interviewing, observing, and inspecting your patient. Then you'll write down the data you've gathered as soon as possible, so you won't forget what you've learned.

As I discuss the items I'll want you to cover, keep this important point in mind: Never document anything without having some idea how it'll help you.

Naturally, you've already determined whether you need a long-term data base on your patient or a short-term one. Find

NURSING DATA BASE
Patient/Family Assessment Guide

◆REASON FOR HOSPITALIZATION OR CHIEF COMPLAINT: As patient sees it.

◆DURATION OF THIS PROBLEM: As patient recalls it, has it affected his life-style?

◆OTHER ILLNESSES AND/OR PREVIOUS EXPERIENCE WITH HOSPITALIZATION: Reason? When? Results? Impressions of previous hospitalizations? Problems encountered? Effect of this hospitalization on education? Family? Child care? Employment? Finances?

◆OBSERVATION OF PATIENT'S CONDITION: Levels of consciousness? Well-nourished? Healthy? Color? Skin turgor? Senses? Headaches? Cough? Syncope? Nausea? Convulsions? Edema? Lumps? Bruises/bleeding? Inflammation? Integrity of skin? Pressure areas? Temperature? Range of motion? Unusual sensations? Paralysis? Odors? Discharges? Pain?

◆MENTAL/EMOTIONAL STATUS: Cooperative? Understanding? Anxiety? Language? Expectations? Feelings about illness? State of consciousness? Mood? Self image? Reaction to stress? Rapport with interviewer/staff? Compatibility with roommate?

◆ALLERGIES: Food? Drugs? Type of reaction?

◆MEDICATION: Dosage? Why taken? When taken? Last dose? Does he have it with him? Any others taken occasionally? Recently? Why? Ask about OTC drugs — i.e., ASA — cough preparations.

◆PROSTHESES: Pacemaker? IPPB? Trach? Drainage tubes? Feeding tube? Catheter? Ostomy appliance? Breast form? Hearing aid? Glasses or contacts? Dentures? Cane? Walker? Brace? False eye? Prosthetic leg? Does he have it with him? Need anything?

REVIEW OF SYSTEMS: See assessment guide.

PATTERNS:
  Hygiene: Dentures? Gums? Teeth? Bath or shower? When?
  Rest/sleep: When? Aids? Difficulties?
  Activity status — Exercise/ambulatory aids: Self care? Ambulatory? Daily exercise?
  Elimination — Bladder — bowel: Patterns? Continent? Frequency? Nocturia? Characteristics of stool/urine? Pain? Discharge? Ostomy? Appliances? Who cares for these? Laxatives? Medications?
  Meals/diet: Feeds self? Diet restrictions (therapeutic and cultural or preferential)? Frequency? Snacks? Allergies? Dislikes? Alcohol? Fad diets?
  Health practices: Breast self-exam? Physical exam? Pap smear? Procto? Smoking? EKG? Annual chest X-ray? Practices related to other conditions patient has, i.e., glaucoma testing, urine reduction, weight control?

LIFE-STYLE: Parent? Family? Number of children? Residence? Occupation? Recreation? Diversion? Interests? Financial status? Religion? Education? Ethnic background?

TYPICAL DAY PROFILE: Have patient describe.

INFORMANT: From whom did you obtain this information? Patient? Family? Old records? Ambulance driver?

◆On every admission.

out how your hospital's policy defines the difference by examining that written policy yourself.

List the patient's chief complaint

Now let's look at the second section of your data base. Here's where you write why the patient was hospitalized. Remember, you'll record the information as the patient sees it. You may even want to use the same words.

SECTION II *   Date _3/1/78_   Time _2⁰⁰ P.M._

Reason for hospitalization or chief complaint: ___*vaginal bleeding - post menopausal*___

Duration of this problem/onset: ___*2 months - 1/78*___

Admitting diagnosis: ___*dysfunctional uterine bleeding*___

Then write down the onset and duration of his problem. You can't effectively plan his care without this information (see Chapter 4). For example, how you treat a patient who's had chest pain for 2 months will differ from how you treat a patient who's had chest pain for 2 hours.

If your patient can't tell you exactly when his problem started, you'll have to jog his memory. Sometimes you can do this by guiding him back in time and relating his problem to other events. When he gives more than one symptom as a chief complaint, *record the onset time for each symptom.* For example, write "inflammation of wrists — 2 months; general fatigue — 3 months."

Looking back to get a health picture

Now you're ready to record data about any previous illnesses the patient may have had, or any past hospitalizations. This information helps you get a total health picture of your patient, on which to build a plan of care.

Previous hospitalizations and illnesses

Date	MD	Where	Type of illness or surgery	Patient reaction
1963	Jones	Memorial Hosp	Appendectomy	pleased "good care"
1960	Jones	Memorial Hosp	Cholecystectomy	upset; pt. had no preop instruction

For example, one reason why you'll ask about other illnesses the patient's had is to see if they'll affect his current problem. This data also gives you a record of any chronic illness and what was done for it.

Urge the patient to be as specific as possible when you fill out this section, especially dates, doctors' names, and the names and locations of hospitals. You may need this information to request old records.

How many times your patient has been hospitalized will also affect your care plans for him. For example, suppose he's never been hospitalized. You know right away that he'll require more reassurance and patient teaching about hospital procedures.

Or suppose he's been hospitalized several times. Find out exactly what kind of effect it had on him. If his experiences have all been negative ones, he'll need special treatment to alleviate his anxiety. Ask what upset him most. Then work out a plan that'll minimize or eliminate that problem. Even if you can't do much about it, you'll at least understand why he's distressed.

What's the patient's background?

Next, examine your patient's family-health history. What illnesses did his mother, father, and close relatives have? Find out the exact details, if you can, and use acceptable abbreviations to record the information in your data base (see example below).

Family health history:

Diabetes *↑ father* Heart *neg* Cancer *sister – uterine* Kidney *neg*

TB *neg* COPD *neg* Asthma *neg* Epilepsy *neg*

Psychiatric *neg* Other *none*

Be particularly alert to data that may relate to the patient's current problem. Pay attention to the level of understanding he shows about certain illnesses; it may provide you with an opportunity for patient teaching.

What's the patient really like?

Take a closer look at the patient's personal habits next. Does he smoke or drink alcohol? If he does, *write down the amount*

FAD DIETS

Many people today are following various diets, sometimes without fully understanding their effect on health, and without having a doctor's supervision. When you assess a new patient's condition, check whether he's on one of these diets. It may be causing some of his symptoms. Here are four of the more popular diets and their possible side effects:

LIQUID-PROTEIN DIET

If your patient's on a liquid-protein diet, he probably eats no food, but drinks approximately 8 oz per day of a liquid-protein mixture. At a caloric intake of 250 to 500 calories per day, his weight loss can be as much as 25 lb per month. He's probably been encouraged to drink 1½ qts of water a day, include vitamin and mineral supplements, and add an extra amount of potassium.

Diet theory:

When the body's deprived of its main source of energy from carbohydrates, it will metabolize some of its own fat and protein as an energy source, resulting in weight loss. The dieter takes a predigested protein supplement to ward off actual starvation.

Side effects:

Strict adherence to this diet may be life-threatening. *No one* should use it without medical supervision. Misuse can result in:
- some breakdown in lean-muscle mass
- psychological stress; fatigue
- ketosis (see opposite page)
- diarrhea or constipation
- recurrent dizziness; brief fainting spells, perhaps with apnea
- muscle cramps
- nausea and flatulence
- dry skin
- low blood-sugar levels
- EKG changes.

ZEN MACROBIOTIC DIET

The patient who follows this diet believes that attaining longevity and peace of mind requires not only meditation but also the adoption of rigid dietary practices. The dieter progresses through stages of purification. Each stage requires a different balance of food products.

Diet theory:

According to this diet's advocates, a balance must exist between *yin* (negative) and *yang* (positive) forces. For example: Sugars and fruits are yin; meats and eggs are yang. Most foods are "too strong" for the body. Rice, however, is the only perfect food, and it's the only ingredient of the diet when purification is reached.

Side effects:

If taken to its extreme, the macrobiotic diet can produce:
- scurvy
- hypoproteinemia
- hypocalcemia
- emaciation, with accompanying loss of kidney function
- anemia
- fatigue, lowered resistance to infectious diseases, heavy vaginal discharges, and, among young pregnant women, a high incidence of low-birthweight babies
- rickets, as well as the above disorders, in children.

VEGETARIAN DIET

As you know, the vegetarian's diet consists of nonflesh foods only. Among dieters, restrictions vary: The lacto (milk) vegetarian's diet includes milk; the lacto-ova vegetarian's diet includes milk and egg products. The lacto-ova vegetarian usually has fewer nutritional risks because of the added source of complete protein.

Diet theory:

Many people do not eat meat because of their religious or ethical beliefs.

Side effects:

Vitamin B_{12} deficiency is common, and may become quite advanced before it's diagnosed. This is because the diet contains adequate amounts of folic acid, which tends to mask symptoms of a B_{12} deficiency. The vegetarian dieter may be unaware of his B_{12} deficiency until irreversible degeneration of his spinal cord has set in. (That occurs only under severe deprivation.) Other symptoms associated with poor use of the diet may include:
- soreness of the tongue
- pernicious anemia
- menstrual irregularity
- paresthesia.

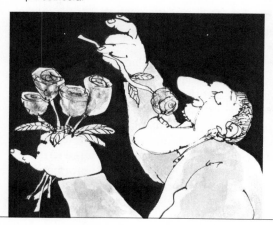

LOW-CARBOHYDRATE DIET

Despite many variations, the common feature of all low-carbohydrate diets is complete elimination of sugar and all-purpose flour, with limitations on other carbohydrate-rich foods: fruit, potatoes, bread, peas, beans, milk, cottage cheese, ice cream, alcohol, etc.

Diet theory:

Supposedly good for hypoglycemia. Advocates contend that low blood sugar is directly associated with fatigue, anxiety, tension, and insomnia.

Side effects:

Because this diet produces ketosis, it may be dangerous for a patient with diabetic tendencies. Restricting carbohydrates also:
- forces the body to excrete large quantities of water, placing stress on the kidneys
- raises the serum-cholesterol level from ingestion of large quantities of meat and dairy products
- increases concentration of uric acid.

This diet sometimes includes large doses of megavitamins, which may lead to skin rashes and kidney problems.

KETOSIS

Ketosis is a condition caused by increased use of the body's fat stores, which are broken down into carbon fragments to be used for energy. However, excess accumulation of these fragments form into ketones, causing ketosis. Ketosis may cause undue strain on the liver and kidney, because ketone bodies are formed in the liver and excreted through the urinary tract. A patient in ketosis also has high levels of uric acid in his bloodstream, which may lead to kidney or bladder stones.

—BARBARA J. KLEEMAN

— for example, 1 pack cigarettes per day; 2 martinis before dinner. This information will help you understand some of the problems he may have when hospitalized, particularly if his habit is now curtailed. It'll forewarn you about the possibility of delirium tremens, if your patient is an alcoholic.

Is your patient allergic to anything? Don't stop at identifying what the substance is. Find out what kind of reaction he had. For example, you'll write "penicillin allergy; reaction: hives, generalized."

Or you may find that your patient just *thinks* he has an allergy to a certain medication because his doctor stopped giving it to him. Check it out. His doctor may have stopped the drug because it wasn't helping, not because it was causing an allergic reaction.

Social history of alcohol *occasional soc. drink* Smoking *1 pack/day*

Allergies (what and type of reaction) *penicillin – severe hives, generalized*

What about medications?

Now let's go on to the section listing the drugs your patient is taking. Make sure you record all essential information. For example, document not only the drug's name, but also the dosage, time routine, last dose prior to admission, and *patient's* reason for why he's taking it.

Sometimes a patient is uncertain about why he's taking a particular drug, which may point up the need for teaching on your part. But it helps to identify the condition for another reason: *You can double-check to make sure you have all his problems listed on your data base.*

Make sure your patient understands that you want him to include over-the-counter preparations. Many patients don't consider these significant. But they'll give you a better understanding of his health habits and perhaps even help you to identify existing problems. Also, a patient may even be causing some of his problems by taking an over-the-counter drug: for example, one that interacts adversely with a prescribed drug he's receiving. Take care to write all the information down, including the amount he's taking and the length of time he's done so.

Medications code: A — Sent home with family; B — May be self-administered;
C — Not brought in with patient.

Name	Code	Dose and Time	Time of last dose	Patient's understanding of purpose
Orinase	C	0.25 g — B.I.D.	5 ^{pm} - 2/28	to treat diabetes

Recording what you've observed and inspected

Soon you've reached that part of the form where you record
your physical assessment findings. Here you'll write exactly
what you've observed and inspected — as you learned how to
do in Chapter 4.

Describe each finding thoroughly. For example, if you write
that a patient has a decubitus ulcer, don't just write where it is.
Record its exact measurements, color, type of drainage, and
odor, if any. Then document if the patient says he feels pain
from that decubitus, or if he says he feels no pain.

Remember, thorough descriptions of all you observe and
inspect are necessary. They provide you with the proper
baseline data you need to measure later improvement or de-
terioration.

Review of systems:

EENT _Conjunctiva pale - PEERLA - nose and throat neg._
pt. denies visual or hearing problems.

Neurological _no problems with ambulation - no_
numbness or paresthesias.

Pulmonary _morning cough that pt. attributes to smoking_
chest clear to auscultation and percussion.

Cardiovascular _B.P. elevated $^{140}/_{100}$ - NSR at 90 - no murmurs_
PMI @ 5 ICS at MCL - no pedal edema - no varicose veins

GI _denies anorexia, nausea, or vomiting - scars in RLQ_
and RUQ from previous surgeries.

GU *no nocturia or frequency - has had UTI x 2 during past 20 years*

Skin *dry - no bruises, scabs or ulcerations noted, no rashes.*

Mental/emotional status *verbalizes concern about bleeding, and teenage son at home.*

Reproductive *Vaginal bleeding for 2 months*

Signature for assessment _____ *M. Reilly, R.N.*

*Must be completed and signed by RN on all admissions

Never use vague terms. For example, don't write that any area of your patient's body looks "normal." What's normal for a patient of one age or condition may not be normal for a patient of another. Furthermore, what's normal to you may not seem normal to another health-team member.

The same applies to the word "negative." If you use the word, be sure you indicate what you're referring to. For example, don't say "negative" next to cardiovascular system. Instead, write "negative for cough, shortness of breath, and chest pain." To merely write the word "negative" leaves too many questions unanswered. It also suggests that you didn't do a complete assessment, or were too uninformed to know what you were looking for.

What's the patient's complaint?
Always remember the patient's chief complaint when you record your findings. Have you shown how it's affecting other areas of his body? Have you listed every function that it does affect and described that effect in detail? For example, suppose your patient has joint pains. Write down all significant findings. Include such things as range-of-motion ability, muscle strength, signs of inflammation, as well as character, extent, and duration of pain.

Describe the patient's life-style
Your patient's personal habits and health patterns will affect his stay in the hospital, especially if he's in for more than 48 hours. So be sure you record what those habits and patterns are so you can plan his care around them.

Consider your patient's personal hygiene habits, for exam-

SECTION III * Date _3/2/78_ Time _11 a.m._

Patterns:

1. Hygiene _bathes nightly_

2. Rest/sleep _requires 8 hours nightly_

3. Activity status _no previous problems with ambulation_

4. Elimination habits _occ. constipation—sees this as no problem, includes roughage in diet_

5. Meals/diet _1800 cal. ADA - occ. uses diabetic candy_

6. Health practices _had yearly pap smear. Sees internist regularly for DM._

Typical daily profile: _up with family at 6³⁰ a.m. Back to bed till nine. Housework, shopping - occasionally plays bridge with friends; spends evenings with family._

ple. Does he regularly take a hot bath before he retires? Will the change of routine upset him if you ask him to shower in the morning?

What about his sleep patterns? Suppose he tells you he regularly works the night shift on his job. Write this information down, so you won't be concerned later when the patient has trouble falling asleep.

Ask him to describe what he eats and drinks during an average day, and record it. This information can be more important than you think, especially if your patient's scheduled for surgery. For example, suppose your patient confides that he's on a fad diet — or regularly drinks 10 to 12 cups of coffee per day. If he's on an unbalanced diet, he may have a serious electrolyte disorder that'll impede his recovery after surgery. If he drinks too much coffee, he'll probably have caffeine-withdrawal headaches on a day he can't drink fluids.

Now record the regular activities your patient pursues when he's healthy. What effect will his illness or impending surgery have on them? Does he understand what he can and cannot do? Will he need a lot of patient teaching? For example, he may not know he can't get up and take his regular shower the morning after surgery. Or he may not realize he's going to tire easily. Describe his normal activities in detail, so you'll know what restrictions you'll have to discuss with him.

Bedside notes for better charting
Some hospitals now place forms for nurses' notes at the patient's bedside. Besides saving time spent on end-of-shift charting, this practice helps make notes more accurate and objective. When a nurse takes a blood pressure reading or gives a p.r.n. medication, she can record it immediately on the notes. The day-shift nurses distribute the forms each morning, the evening-shift nurses pick them up during their last rounds, and the night-shift nurses record them on the patient charts. Where are they usually kept? Under the activity flow sheets, on a clipboard at the foot of the bed.

Make notes about his bowel and bladder habits. Does he take a daily laxative? If he does, you'll have to place an order for a laxative, or your patient's routine will be upset. You may also want to include some patient teaching in his care to warn him of the hazards of frequent laxative use. And you'll probably ask the dietician to visit him so he knows what foods aid regular elimination.

Documenting how many times a night the patient says he gets up to void is also important. It may even prevent a serious accident from happening, as you recall from the story at the beginning of this chapter.

If your patient's a woman, ask about her menstrual history. But don't just say, "Is it normal?" Encourage her to relate specific information: For example, has it changed in any way and does she take any medications before or during her period? Pay attention to the words she uses to describe menstruation. If her education is weak in this area, she may need some patient teaching. She may also need additional tests to determine the cause of any difficulties she's having.

Record as much information as you can about your patient's health practices. Determine what kind of emphasis he places on regular care. For example, does he have a regular checkup? If the patient is a woman, does she examine her breasts at least once a month?

If you detect that your patient is careless about his health, make plans to educate him. Document the words he uses to describe his body functions, so you can gear your patient teaching to his level.

In short, you want a complete picture — in writing — of your patient's personal habits and life-style. You may find this time-consuming to record, but you'll need it to build an effective care plan.

One quick way to make sure you have that complete picture is to ask for a typical day profile. Have the patient describe it in his own words and encourage him to relate as many details as he feels are necessary.

You may be surprised at the information you gather when you ask about a typical day. For example, you may find that the patient doesn't have a typical day. He may have an unusual schedule that makes every day of the week different. You need to know this because it can affect his condition. He may find it difficult to take his medication on schedule when he's discharged, or he may not have time for the routine self-care he needs.

But "typical day" information is valuable to you for another reason. It may help you determine why the patient was hospitalized. For example. I heard about a young diabetic's difficulty in getting his condition controlled. When an alert nurse asked him to describe a typical day, he told her about his unusual schedule for school and work. As a result, he couldn't always fit in his prescribed diet and he sometimes skipped his morning insulin because he slept late.

So you see, documenting all these facts about a patient helps you build effective care plans for him. Not only care plans for use while he's hospitalized, but care plans to follow when he's discharged. If you neglect to get the information you need, you'll find it out haphazardly. Or you won't find it out at all, which may ultimately prove disastrous.

The final step
Now you've reached the end of the initial assessment form, which you'll see in its entirety in Chapter 6. Indicate who gave you the information or where you got it. Remember to record significant information that came with your patient from other hospitals, particularly if he's being transferred. By indicating where you got the facts you recorded, you make it easier to go back to the source and check it. You enable yourself and others to obtain additional information about the patient, if it's necessary.

Information obtained from:

Patient ___✓___ Family _____ Previous records _____

COMMENTS: _patient expects to have surgery in near future and is concerned about teenage son at home — blood pressure is elevated at this time, which requires further assessment. pt. verbalizes a good understanding of diabetes and its control._

Signature _____ M. Reilly, R.N. _____
*Completed by an RN for long-term admissions only

Soon you'll start reading the next chapters and learn how to write care plans based on your initial assessment. Before you do, review these tips on how to document:

Remember these rules about documenting your initial assessment:

1. Always document your initial assessment as soon as possible after you interview, observe, and inspect.

2. Always document your assessment *away* from the patient's bedside. Jot down only key points while you're with the patient.

3. Always answer every question on the assessment form. If a question doesn't apply to your patient, write "N/A" or "not applicable" in the space.

4. Always focus your questions on areas that relate to the patient's chief complaint. Record information that has *significance* and will help you build a care plan.

5. If you delegate the job of filling out the first section of the form to another nurse, LPN, or aide, remember this: You *must* review the information gathered and validate it if you're not sure it's correct.

6. Always accept accountability for your assessment by signing your name to the areas you've completed.

7. Always directly quote the patient or family member who gave you the information, if you fear that summarizing will make it lose some of its meaning.

8. Always write or print legibly, in ink.

9. Always be concise, specific, and exact when you describe your physical findings.

10. Always go back to the patient's bedside to clarify or validate information that seems incomplete.

SKILLCHECK 2

1. As you approach 19-year-old Jane Simmons, a newly-arrived patient, to interview her, she suddenly bursts into tears. How should you react?
a) Leave Jane alone to gain composure before you interview her.
b) Apologize to Jane for disturbing her; explain that it is necessary to interview her at this time.
c) Ask Jane if she would prefer that you come back later.
d) Show Jane you are concerned and willing to listen if she chooses to discuss her problem with you.

2. During an interview, 62-year-old Arthur Samuels confides that he occasionally has breathing problems. What do you say next?
a) "Tell me more about these problems."
b) "Do you mean you have a cough?"
c) "Smoking may have contributed to your problems."
d) "Do you have heart problems that you know of?"

3. You're interviewing Jim Walker, a 29-year-old bricklayer, when the maintenance man arrives to repair an empty bed in the room. He explains that the work must be done before the bed's usual occupant returns from physical therapy. What do you do?
a) Ask the maintenance man to return later.
b) Tell Mr. Walker you will return later.
c) Draw the curtain and ask Mr. Walker to ignore the noise.
d) Complete the interview in a quieter area.

4. Hannah King, a 34-year-old housewife, absolutely refuses to discuss her husband's reaction to her recent mastectomy. What do you say?
a) Tell Mrs. King it's okay because you will be talking to her husband about this anyway.
b) Insist that this information is important to her care plan.
c) Convince her that she should discuss this matter freely because you will keep it confidential.
d) Reassure her that she has a right not to reveal this information.

5. The time you've allotted to interview Roger Ferris is up and he's answered all your questions. What is the *next* step you should take?
a) Thank Mr. Ferris for his help and return to the nurse's station to begin writing a care plan.
b) Inform him that the interview is completed and you will return later.
c) Ask him how *he* sees his problems, summarize your findings, and together work out possible solutions.
d) Conclude the interview by informing him that you will use the information to plan effective nursing care.

6. Latonya Gaskin, a 28-year-old waitress, has just been admitted to your unit. Give one reason why you'd document her usual pattern of daily living.
a) to alter those habits which don't fit hospital routine
b) to alter those habits not considered typical
c) to plan care according to established habits
d) to analyze personality traits.

7. You notice that Marcia Staver, a 24-year-old newly arrived patient, answers your questions in a very hoarse voice. What do you do first?
a) Question her about its beginning and duration.
b) Observe and culture her throat; palpate cervical lymph nodes.
c) Anticipate a long-term problem and suggest non-verbal means of communication.
d) Notify the doctor.

8. During your initial assessment of Harry Stein, a 48-year-old garment worker, he tells you that he's in the hospital for a checkup because he's been feeling tired lately. You know the doctor's admitting diagnosis is cancer of the colon. What do you write under "reason for hospitalization"?
a) cancer of the colon
b) possible anemia due to gastrointestinal cancer
c) diagnostic evaluation
d) "to have a good checkup because I have been feeling tired lately."

9. Which of the following documentations of physical assessment findings is the most accurate and thorough?
a) EENT: *No complaint of earache or discharge*
b) Pulmonary: *Respiratory system appears normal*
c) GI: *Appetite good, liver not enlarged*
d) GU: *Negative for frequency, nocturia, pain, hematuria, discharge.*

(Answers on page 180)

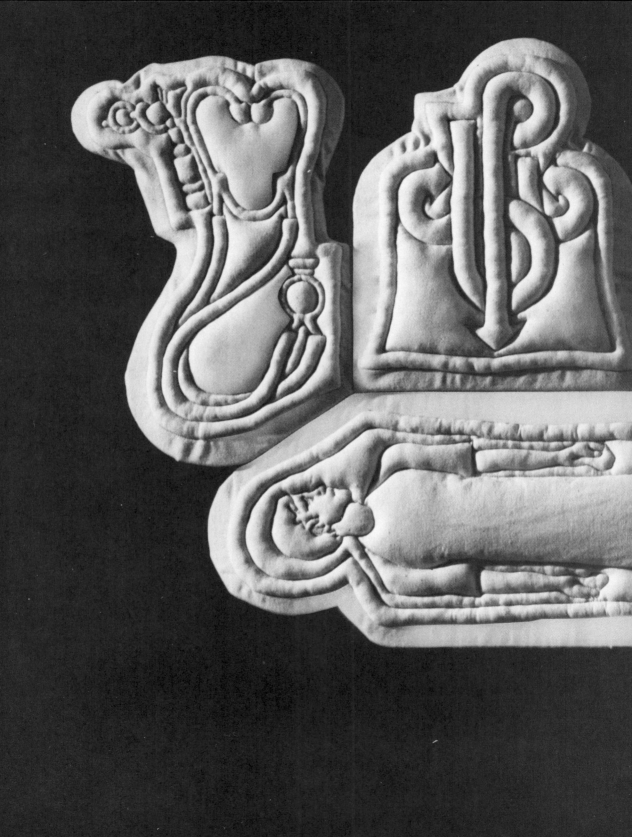

HOW TO IDENTIFY
YOUR PATIENT'S PROBLEMS
AND PLAN HIS CARE

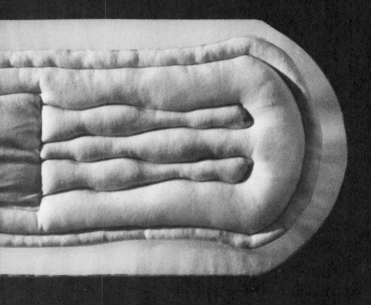

"A problem is any condition or situation
  that a patient
  can't readily handle himself —
  one that requires intervention by you
  or some other member of the health-care team."

"Always identify the patient's problems
  at the level you know they exist."

"Your care plan shows everyone
  the goals you've set
  for your patient and gives clear directions
  for helping him achieve those goals."

"When you write a care plan, be specific;
  don't use vague terms or generalities."

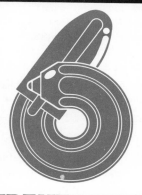

IDENTIFYING YOUR PATIENT'S PROBLEMS
Which ones need attention

BY MARY M. REILLY, RN, BSN

JUST 6 DAYS AFTER he arrived in the U.S. on a vacation trip, French-speaking Jean-Paul Saulnier had an acute myocardial infarction. He was rushed to the emergency department of a nearby hospital, where he received effective initial treatment for his condition.

Later in the CCU, the head nurse reviewed his assessment data, identified his problems, and wrote out his care plans. Had the nurse been less skilled at this task, she might have overlooked one of these problems. Monsieur Saulnier couldn't speak English, which immediately created a communication barrier between him and members of the health-care team.

Have trouble identifying problems?
Just what is a problem? Which ones require care plans? How many do you list for each patient? And are they *his* problems or *yours*? Suppose you have a confirmed medical diagnosis to work with? Do you list that as the patient's only physical problem? Or do you list his *symptoms* as problems so you can deal with each independently?

If you're uncertain about all this, you'll find the answers in

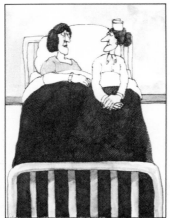

From the patient's perspective
Caring for your patients can make
their problems seem like your
problems. But in the truest sense,
problems are difficulties or
concerns experienced by the
patient. Writing a good care plan
requires learning to see problems
from the perspective of the patient
and his family.
  Finding the answers to these
questions will help you express
problems in terms of the patient's
perspective:
  • What's happening to the
patient physiologically?
  • What clinical signs is he
manifesting?
  • What's happening to him
emotionally, socially, or
spiritually?
  • How does the patient — and
his family — feel about what's
happening?
  • How are they coping with the
situation?

this chapter. I'll explain exactly how to write a problem list for
your problem-oriented record, so you won't have any trouble
formulating your care plans.

Suppose you use the source-oriented system. Then you
don't write a formal problem list, as you know. But you'll still
gain insight from this chapter on how to identify your patient's
problems.

What are problems anyway?
Think back to our explanation of the nursing process (Chapter 1). Remember how it relates to the standard method
of problem-solving? As a nurse, you must:

• Observe and recognize your patient's problems (assessment).

• Define each problem specifically (problem identification
and nursing diagnosis).

• Arrive at possible solutions for each problem (care planning).

• Put those solutions to work (implementation).

• Determine if those solutions were successful (evaluation).

Completing Step 2 is crucial, as you can see. You can't
effectively care for your patient unless you identify his problems. You can't even document his progress properly, because you have nothing specific to relate that progress to.

But what *is* a problem? I like this definition: A problem is
any condition or situation that a patient can't readily handle
himself — one that requires intervention by you or some other
member of the health-care team. Since you must always view
the patient as a whole person, you'll consider more than just
his physical complaints. For example, you may identify a
problem like this: "Patient can't buy needed medications after
discharge because he lacks money."

In other words, you can correctly identify one of the
patient's financial or emotional *needs* as a problem, if it interferes with his well-being. You can also identify a *symptom* as a
problem: for example, incontinence, vomiting, or vaginal
bleeding.

Can you identify a medical diagnosis as a problem? Yes, if
the doctor's *confirmed* it. Never write down a suspected medical diagnosis. Start at the symptom level and *list problems
only as you know they exist*.

For example, suppose a patient comes into the hospital with

hyperglycemia. And you know the doctor suspects diabetes mellitus. You don't write diabetes mellitus at that point. You just write hyperglycemia.

Don't even write "possible" diabetes as a problem. Stay with existing symptoms. List the medical diagnosis as a problem later, when and if it's confirmed.

Don't standardize

I want you to remember a few other general rules about identifying your patient's problems. Don't attempt to standardize them too much. *Remember no problem can be exactly the same for each patient, because each patient is an individual.*

For example, you may have two patients who need to be taught how to stay on identical low-fat diets, but one lives with his son and daughter-in-law. That patient doesn't prepare his own meals, so your care plan will have to include a teaching session for his family.

Remember potential problems

List a potential problem, if it's likely to occur. Then you'll have a special care plan ready when you need it. For example, if you know an alcoholic patient may get delirium tremens after 4 days without alcohol (even with preventative measures), get orders and plan how to restrain him.

Sometimes, you can even prevent a problem from occurring by identifying it. For instance, you might label skin breakdown a potential problem for an elderly patient with a fractured hip. Then you'd write a care plan that included regular turning for him, as well as other preventative measures.

Potential problems sometimes become obvious when you review data about the patient's typical day. For example, suppose you know your diabetic patient has an unusual work schedule. You'll give him special help before and at discharge to arrange his meal times to fit his insulin therapy.

Doing it the problem-oriented way

Now, let's examine the problem-oriented system of writing a problem list. As you know, you write this on a separate sheet, listing not only active problems (acute and chronic), but past problems, as well.

To understand exactly how problems are written on the complete problem-oriented list, let's imagine you're caring for

Identifying problems

Here are some examples of common types of problems:
- A specific diagnosis or syndrome, e.g., peptic ulcer, thoracic outlet syndrome
- A sign or symptom, e.g., ascites, fever
- An abnormal laboratory value, e.g., hyperkalemia
- An operation, e.g., status post-appendectomy
- An allergy or risk factor, e.g., iodine allergy, obesity
- A psychological or social problem, e.g., fear of suffocation, no one to care for children, unemployment
- A demographic problem, e.g., asbestos exposure
- An incomplete data base.

a 52-year-old patient named Elizabeth Tanner, who's just been admitted to your unit with severe vaginal bleeding. (See her completed assessment form in this chapter.)

During your interview, observation, and inspection, you find out that Mrs. Tanner's bleeding began 2 months earlier, and just recently increased in amount. When you question her about her menstrual history, you learn that she is post-menopausal. So you write this information on your problem list as I've illustrated below, showing the month and year the problem began. Be sure to sign your name opposite the entry, so other members of the health-care team know who originally identified the problem.

Date onset	No.	Active problems (acute and chronic)	Name	Date resolved	Inactive or resolved problems
01/78	1	vaginal bleeding – post menopausal	M. Reilly RN		

Since the cause of Mrs. Tanner's vaginal bleeding is not known at this time, leave a few lines blank — so you can update the problem with new information later.

Nursing tip: Draw a heavy red line below the last blank line to indicate to others that you want the space above it saved. Then no one will write in *another* problem in the space you're saving to resolve the first one.

As you review the rest of the data you've collected about Mrs. Tanner, you identify several other problems — all of which seem worthy of an entry on your problem list.

Date onset	No.	Active problems (acute and chronic)	Name	Date resolved	Inactive or resolved problems
1955	2	obesity, adult onset	M. Reilly RN		
	3	⟶	M. Reilly RN	1953	appendectomy
	4	⟶	M. Reilly RN	1960	cholecystectomy
1958	5	diabetes mellitus	M. Reilly RN		
1960	6	allergy to penicillin	M. Reilly RN		
3/2/78	7	concern over teenage son at home	M. Reilly RN		
3/2/78	8	elevated BP – systolic & diastolic	M. Reilly RN		

Problems 3 and 4, as you can see, were resolved years before you assessed Mrs. Tanner. When you identify a *resolved* problem, you draw an arrow leading to that problem in the Inactive or Resolved column.

This probably brings a question to mind: How do you know which resolved problems to list? Obviously, you can't list every minor fracture or illness that's occurred throughout the patient's life. Try to list those that seem significant, or in some way related to the patient's active problems. If you're *in doubt* about a resolved problem, enter it just to be safe.

Problem 8, which is Mrs. Tanner's elevated blood pressure, is something you noticed during your initial inspection. But, you haven't diagnosed the cause of the problem — or even called it hypertension — you've only identified it as you see it. Later, if the *doctor* identifies Mrs. Tanner's problem as hypertension, you can update this entry on your list. Leave a few lines blank at this spot, and draw a red line so no one writes in the space.

Now, let's go back to Problem 1 — Mrs. Tanner's vaginal bleeding. Two days after she's admitted to the hospital, she has a dilation and curretage (D and C), and the doctor diagnoses a fibroid uterus. You enter this new information next to your original note about vaginal bleeding in this way, using an arrow with a date above it to indicate progression.

Date onset	No.	Active problems (acute and chronic)	Name	Date resolved	Inactive or resolved problems
01/78	1	vaginal bleeding - post menopausal _3-3-78 D&C → Fibroid uterus_	M. Reilly RN		

After consulting with her doctor, Mrs. Tanner decides to have a total hysterectomy, and two days later the surgery is performed. This information is still related to her original problem of vaginal bleeding, so you enter it under Problem 1 in this way:

Date onset	No.	Active problems (acute and chronic)	Name	Date resolved	Inactive or resolved problems
01/78	1	vaginal bleeding - post menopausal _3-3-78 D&C Fibroid uterus 3-5-78 total abd. hysterectomy_	M. Reilly RN	3/14/78	

NURSING DATA BASE
(Assessment)

SECTION I: Date _3/1/78_ Time _1³⁰ p.m._ Name _Elizabeth Tanner_

Mode _Ambulatory_ Age _52_

T _99⁶_ P _90_ R _18_ BP _140/100_ Ht _5'3"_ Wt _156_

Diet _1800 cal. ADA_ Bloodwork: Yes _✓_ No _____ Urinalysis: Yes _✓_ No _____

Prosthesis: Glasses _none_ Contact lenses _none_ Dentures _none_ Other _none_

General orientation to hospital environment by: _M. Adams, LPN_ _3/1/78_
Signature / Date

Section I must be completed and signed by an RN or LPN on all admissions.

SECTION II: Date _3/1/78_ Time _2⁰⁰ P.M._

Reason for hospitalization or chief complaint: _vaginal bleeding - post menopausal_

Duration of this problem/onset: _2 months 1/78_

Admitting diagnosis: _dysfunctional uterine bleeding_

Previous hospitalizations and illnesses:

Date	MD	Where	Type of illness or surgery and reaction
1963	Jones	Memorial Hosp.	Appendectomy — no problems
1960	Jones	Memorial Hosp.	Cholecystectomy — upset - no preop instruction

Family Health History:

Diabetes _↑ father_ Heart _neg_ Cancer _sister uterine_ Kidney _neg_ T.B. _neg_ COPD _neg_

Asthma _neg_ Epilepsy _neg_ Psychiatric _neg_ Other _none_

Social history of alcohol _occ. soc. drink_ Smoking _1 pack cigarettes/day_

Allergies (what and type of reaction) _penicillin - severe hives, generalized_

Medications code: A — Sent home with family; B — May be self-administered; C — Not brought in with patient.

Name	Code	Dose and time	Time of last dose	Patient's understanding of purpose
Orinase	C	0.25 g - B.I.D	5 P.M. 2/28	to treat diabetes

Review of Systems:

EENT _Conjunctiva pale - PEERLA - nose and throat neg; pt. denies visual or hearing problems_

Neurological _no problems with ambulation - no numbness or paresthesias_

Pulmonary _morning cough that pt. attributes to smoking. Chest clear to auscultation and percussion_

Cardiovascular _B.P. elevated ¹⁴⁰/₁₀₀ - NSR at 90 - no murmurs PMI @ 5 ICS at MCL - no pedal edema - no varicose veins_

GI _denies anorexia, nausea or vomiting - scars in RLQ & RUQ_
from previous surgeries

GU _no nocturia or frequency - has had UTI x 2 during_
past 20 years

Skin _dry - no bruises, scabs or ulcerations noted,_
no rashes

Mental/emotional status _verbalizes concern about bleeding and teenage son at home_

Reproductive _vaginal bleeding for 2 months_

Signature for minimal assessment _M. Reilly, RN_

Section II must be completed and signed by an RN (both Sections I and II must be completed on short-term admissions).

SECTION III: Date _3/2/78_   Time _11 AM_

Patterns:

Hygiene _bathes nightly_

Rest/sleep _requires 8 hours nightly_

Activity status _no previous problems with ambulation_

Elimination habits _occ. constipation - sees this as no problem; include roughage in diet_

Meals/diet _1800 cal. ADA - occ. uses diabetic candy_

Health practices _has yearly pap smear. Sees internist regularly for DM_

Typical daily profile: _up with family at 6³⁰ a.m. Back to bed till 9⁰⁰_
housework, shopping - occasionally plays bridge with friends
spends evenings with family

Information obtained from: Patient _✓_ Family _____ Previous records _____

COMMENTS: _Patient expects to have surgery in near future and is_
concerned about teenage son at home. Blood pressure is elevated at
this time which requires further assessment. Pt. verbalizes a
good understanding of diabetes and its control.

Signature _M. Reilly, RN_

Section III — Completed by an RN. (Sections I, II and III must be completed on all patients except those defined by policy as short-term.)

SECTION IV: Date _____   Time _____

Review and update on readmissions (include vital signs & positive findings of system review).

COMMENTS: _____ TPR _____ BP _____

not applicable

Signature _____

Section IV — Completed by RN on patients defined by policy as readmissions.

Remember, as new problems arise for your patient, you must add them to your list. For example, let's imagine Mrs. Tanner develops a fever 3 days postop. Since her wound looks clean and dry with no signs of infection, and her lungs are clear, the doctor orders a urine culture and sensitivity. Mrs. Tanner may have developed a urinary tract infection from the Foley catheter she had in place for 24 hours postop.

You'd enter Mrs. Tanner's fever as Problem 9, noting the date of onset. Then you'd list the results of the diagnostic procedure as indicated below:

Date onset	No.	Active problems (acute and chronic)	Name	Date resolved	Inactive or resolved problems
3/8/78	9	Fever, postop $\xrightarrow{\text{3-10-78}}$ C+S urinary tract infection	M. Reilly RN	3/14/78	

Your diagnosis and the doctor's: Finding a place for both
Remember how the term "nursing diagnosis" was explained in Chapter 1. Your nursing diagnosis identifies any problem that interferes with your patient's well-being. You never diagnose the *cause* of a medical problem. That responsibility belongs to the doctor.

So what do you do with a medical diagnosis when it's finally confirmed? Where does it fit on your problem list? Some nurses have trouble deciding. Because, up to that point, they've been concentrating only on their nursing diagnoses.

However, never go to such extreme that you write only the problems *you've* identified on the patient's chart. A confirmed medical diagnosis must always be listed as a patient problem.

Confirmed or not confirmed
A good rule to follow is this: List symptoms as separate problems until you get a confirmed medical diagnosis. Then — when you get the medical diagnosis — update the symptoms, as I'll illustrate on the next page, using the problem-oriented system.

For example, suppose a patient comes to the hospital with these symptoms: edema, productive cough, and dyspnea. Since you don't have a confirmed medical diagnosis to go with these problems, you'll list them as follows:

Date onset	No.	Active problems (acute and chronic)	Name	Date resolved	Inactive or resolved problems
5/23/78	1	Edema	J. Kraft RN		
	2	Productive cough	J. Kraft RN		
	3	Dyspnea	J. Kraft RN		

Now, imagine that the doctor writes a confirmed medical diagnosis of congestive heart failure for this same patient. You'd update your problem list by adding the information in this fashion:

Date onset	No.	Active problems (acute and chronic)	Name	Date resolved	Inactive or resolved problems
5/23/78	1	Edema → secondary to CHF	J. Kraft RN		
	2	Productive cough → combine c̄ #1	J. Kraft RN		
	3	Dyspnea → combine c̄ #1	J. Kraft RN		

The arrows show that you now understand your patient's symptoms on a higher level. You've combined them and now refer to them as one problem with one number.

Suppose, however, this patient we're talking about already *has* a confirmed diagnosis of congestive heart failure. Don't number his symptoms as individual, unrelated problems as you did in my first example. Take the number the doctor has given his recorded diagnosis and list the related symptoms under it, as I illustrate below:

Date onset	No.	Active problems (acute and chronic)	Name	Date resolved	Inactive or resolved problems
5/23/78	1	Congestive heart failure	J. Kraft RN		
	1A	Edema	J. Kraft RN		
	1B	Productive cough	J. Kraft RN		
	1C	Dyspnea	J. Kraft RN		

Keep it practical

Now, won't this method of listing symptoms underneath each diagnosis become unwieldy? It can, if you don't use common sense when you use it. Don't list every symptom that relates to

Tips on writing nursing goals

When you write goals, always start with a specific action verb that focuses on the patient's behavior. Why? Because by telling your reader how your patient should *look, walk, eat, drink, turn, cough, speak, stand,* etc., you give a clear picture by which to evaluate his progress.

Get rid of unnecessary words; make your writing more concise. For example, don't begin your goals with the phrase "The patient will..." If the goal's for the patient, you've stated the obvious. Specify which person the goal is for only where family, friends, or others are directly concerned.

Avoid starting goal statements with *allow, let, enable,* or similar verbs. Such words focus attention on your own and other health-team members' behavior, *not* on the patient's.

a confirmed medical diagnosis; *list only those that are major management problems.*

For example, suppose your patient with congestive heart failure has pitting edema. You wouldn't list the edema as a separate problem; you'd deal with it as part of congestive heart failure. However, suppose that edema doesn't respond to diuretics and keeps your patient from walking. List it as a separate problem related to the diagnosis, and write a specific care plan.

Nursing tip: Never lump your patient's problems together so much that you can't write any care plan. But never split them up so much that your problem list becomes unwieldy.

Do you identify problems on a Kardex care plan?

In the source-oriented system, your patients' problems are identified *only* on the Kardex. *It becomes the only tool you have for planning patient care.*

In the true problem-oriented system, however, the Kardex isn't really essential, because the patient's problem list and *initial* plan are part of his chart (see Chapter 2).

Still, some hospitals using POMR feel that the Kardex is a worthwhile organizational tool and copy the initial plan on it anyway. Others compromise the system still further and write the initial plan directly on the Kardex, instead of keeping it separate in the chart. Then after discharge, this Kardex becomes a part of the patient's permanent record.

No matter what system or combination of systems you have in your hospital, if you write problems on a *Kardex* you need to know how to do it effectively.

Coping with the Kardex

As you can see from the example below, the usual Kardex shows just two columns in which to write problems, goals, and approaches (nursing orders).

Date	Patient problems and goals	Approach (nursing order)

Ideally, your Kardex should show a total of six columns, as

I've illustrated below. You may want to revise yours by adding lines and headings with your pen and ruler.

CARE PLAN

Date	D/C'd date	Problem	Goal	Target date	Approach (nursing orders)

*If you use POMR, add still another column for the problem number.

Now, you're ready to list your patient's problems on the Kardex. Try to do this as soon as possible after the patient's admission and follow these important steps:

• Review all the data you've collected during your initial assessment. Take at least as much time *thinking* about that data and its significance as you did *collecting* it.

• Consider the problem category list on page 81. This will help you identify *all* the patient's problems, not just his physical ones.

• If you have trouble identifying the patient's problems even after you've systematically reviewed his assessment, go back to his *symptoms* and decide if any are major problems. *Never leave a problem blank because you're unsure of what to write.*

• Write down the goals you want your patient to reach with your help. Select a goal for each problem and record a target date for each goal to be accomplished.

Setting your goals
Let me explain what I mean by a nursing goal. You'll never know if you solved your patient's problem without one. You have to know exactly how you want your patient to respond to your care before you can arrive at a workable plan.

To do this, imagine what you want your patient to *do*, how you want him to *look*, or what you want him to *say*. Then state that goal clearly and specifically next to each problem on your list.

For example, if the doctor has diagnosed your patient's problem as emphysema, don't write that your goal is to "improve the patient's respiratory functioning." Be specific. Write exactly how you want the patient to respond to your care: For example, "Patient will show no dyspnea or cyanosis after ambulating for 15 minutes."

Along with each goal, you must list a realistic target date for that goal to be reached. Be flexible enough to adjust that date if your patient needs more time to respond to your care plan. But always set a target date, so you can discontinue a care plan if it's not working and write another that will be more effective. (For complete details on how to write individualized care plans for your patients, read Chapters 7 and 8.)

Based on what I've told you so far, you'd write your patient's problems on the Kardex care plan like this — allowing space, of course, after each one to fill out your nursing approach.

CARE PLAN

Date	D/C'd date	Problem	Goal	Target date	Approach (nursing orders)
4/8/78		#1 Emphysema	Patient will show no dyspnea or cyanosis p̄ ambulating for 15 mins.	4/22/78	

What about new problems?

Anytime new problems arise, add them to your problem list or the patient's care plan on the Kardex. Be sure to indicate that a problem's discontinued or resolved when your approach has accomplished its goal. In this way, you give yourself and others a clear picture of your patient's condition every time you look at his problem list or Kardex care plan.

Summing up

Regardless of which system — or combination of systems you use — identifying your patient's problems *correctly* is what really counts. Accurate problem identification is an essential step toward writing a complete and effective patient care plan.

To review what you've learned in this chapter, read the rules on page 92.

DESIGNING HOSPITAL FORMS

If you've ever had to fill out a poorly-designed hospital form, then you know how such a form can turn a simple routine into a demanding chore. As a nurse, you may be asked to join a committee to revise some of the forms used by your hospital. Given the opportunity, could you design a form that would be easy to read and convenient to use?

These suggestions from Nursing Skillbooks' designers and editors can help you:

Decide on the form's purpose. Then make sure that everything on it contributes in some way to that purpose. Remember, a well-designed form works like a machine, helping you to collect and organize information efficiently.

After you've decided on the contents, your next step is to plan a layout. First, arrange all information in a logical sequence. Then determine how much space nurses will need in order to fill out each section properly. This is an important step. Why? Because without sufficient room to write, some of the staff members using the form will make inadequate entries.

A good way to avoid all design problems is to do a field test: Give several nurses copies of the preliminary draft. Ask them to try it out. Then get their reactions before you finalize the form for general use.

On the sample form below we've illustrated some practical tips on layout and typography. Use them when you specify your requirements to the printer.

Capital letters get attention, but a combination of capitals and lower case (small) letters is more legible. Use capitals sparingly.

Allow 3/16" to 1/4" between write-in lines.

If forms will be bound in a loose-leaf binder, allow 5/8" before the left margin.

You may wish to use a heavier ruled line to separate main sections.

Use boldface (heavy) type for section headings.

NURSING DATA BASE
(Assessment)

Section I: Date _____   Time

Mode _____

Diet _____   Bloodwork: Yes _____ No _____

Prosthesis: Glasses _____   Contact lenses _____   Dent

General orientation to hospital environment by: _____

Section II: Date _____   Tim

Reason for hospitalization or chief complaint: _____

Type is measured in *points*. Here are some sample typefaces and their point sizes. Most forms-printing houses have sizes up to 48 point.

SANS SERIF TYPE	SERIF TYPE
12 point Helvetica Bold	**12 point Times Roman Bold**
12 point Helvetica Light	12 point Times Roman
11 point Helvetica Bold	**11 point Times Roman Bold**
11 point Helvetica Light	11 point Times Roman
10 point Helvetica Bold	**10 point Times Roman Bold**
10 point Helvetica Light	10 point Times Roman
9 point Helvetica Bold	**9 point Times Roman Bold**
9 point Helvetica Light	9 point Times Roman
8 point Helvetica Bold	**8 point Times Roman Bold**
8 point Helvetica Light	8 point Times Roman
7 point Helvetica Bold	**7 point Times Roman Bold**
7 point Helvetica Light	7 point Times Roman
6 point Helvetica Bold	**6 point Times Roman Bold**
6 point Helvetica Light	6 point Times Roman

Remember these ten rules when you identify patient problems:

1. **Always** review the patient's data base or assessment guide thoroughly before you identify his problems to insure that no problem or need is overlooked.
2. **Always** consider each category of problems as you review the data base.
3. **Always** identify the patient's problems as soon as possible after the initial assessment.
4. **Always** identify problems at the level you know they exist.
5. **Never** identify a medical or psychiatric diagnosis, unless it has been written on the medical record by a doctor.
6. **Never** write the terms "possible," "probable," or "rule out" in front of a diagnosis.
7. **Always** write a clear, specific *patient* goal for each identified problem.
8. **Always** set a realistic target date for that goal to be reached.
9. **Always** keep your problem list current by adding new problems as they occur, and discontinuing resolved ones.
10. **Never** forget *why* problem identification is important: You must define your patient's problems clearly and specifically before you can find workable solutions for them.

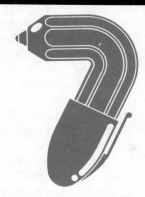

WRITING YOUR PATIENT'S CARE PLAN
How to do it efficiently

BY ELLEN K. VASEY, RN, MPH

"SOMETHING FOR THE Joint Commission…" That's how some nurses regard care plans. Or worse, they think of them as something to write for their supervisor: specifically, extra *paper work* for which they have no time.

I even heard one nurse question the importance of care plans. Why? Because, in her hospital, they were always written in pencil and erased as they were revised. Another nurse complained that everyone *told* her to write care plans, but no one ever explained exactly *how*.

How do *you* react?
What reaction do you get when you hear the term "patient care plans"? Do you know *how* to write them? Do you know *why* you write them — and *what* they accomplish?

In this chapter, I'll answer these questions, so you'll understand this part of the nursing process thoroughly. I'll also give examples of problems that *could've been avoided* with a proper care plan. Then you can better see why they're important.

Remember your role
Obviously, care plans aren't written just to please your super-

In other words
What we call *approaches* are sometimes called *nursing orders*. Both terms refer to the part of a care plan that's tailored to fit a particular patient at a particular time. Develop the approach from a review of the patient's assessment data, and always apply it with a specific goal in mind.

visor or to satisfy the Joint Commission. But before you can really understand *why* they're written, you must first know your role as a nurse.

Your role is to provide quality care for each patient, and you can't do that *unless you plan and direct it*. You must set goals for each patient, so you — and other staff members — know what you hope to accomplish. Never let it be said that a patient recovered *in spite of your care*. Let your well-planned care be the *reason* why he recovered.

You wouldn't think of caring for a patient without *medical* orders. Medical orders are essential. Well, *nursing* orders are also essential. They're just as important to you as medical orders are to the doctor.

So keep reminding yourself about your role as a nurse. Besides assessing your patient and identifying his problems, you must plan, direct, implement, and evaluate his care. If you don't write a care plan after your initial assessment, you've neglected an important step. You've failed to *give direction* to your nursing care, which inevitably affects implementation and evaluation.

How care plans help
A care plan that's well conceived and properly written helps you in many ways. For example, it:
• gives direction to patient care
• establishes continuity of care
• provides a means of communication between you and nurses on other shifts, between you and health-team members in other departments, and between you and your patient
• serves as a key for patient-care assignments.

Giving direction
I've already explained one of the ways a care plan gives direction. It shows everyone the goals you've set for your patient and gives clear directions for helping him achieve them.

But a well-written care plan gives direction in another way: It shows everyone *exactly what to document* on the patient's progress notes. For example, it lists:
• what observations to make and how often
• what nursing measures to take and how to implement them
• what to teach the patient and/or his family before he's discharged.

Using this list as a guideline, you immediately know the specific information you must document. If you have *no* care plan — or a *poorly written* one — you'll never be quite sure what to document.

Providing continuity

Now, let's discuss how a care plan provides continuity of care — even though hospital shift routines change several times each day. First, your care plan identifies the patient's needs to each of those shifts, and tells what must be done for those needs. With this information, nurses on each shift can make their routines fit the patient's care plan — instead of doing it the wrong way: making the patient's care plan fit their routines.

A care plan achieves continuity in still another way: by providing each shift with explicit instructions on how to care for each patient. For example, suppose the patient has gastrointestinal bleeding and requires Maalox, given every 2 hours. A well-written care plan says more than just "Maalox, q 2 hours." It says "Maalox, q 2 hours (even hours)." With this specific instruction, no confusion will exist between shifts, and the patient's care will have continuity.

What happens when your patient's discharged from the hospital? Will his care be turned over to a visiting nurse? Or will he be transferred to another hospital: for example, a nursing home or rehabilitation center? Make sure a copy of his care plan gets transferred with him, so the new health-care team knows what you've been doing. Then your patient's care will retain its continuity, and his transition to the new hospital or nurse will be easier.

A way to communicate

All these points, of course, illustrate how care plans help you *communicate* with other members of the health-care team. But never assume those plans are fulfilling this important function; review them with the other nurses during change-of-shift reports.

By reviewing care plans, you can discuss the patient's response or lack-of-response to the care he's receiving — as well as his medical regime. However, always review as many of those plans with the patient as possible before you discuss them with the other nurses, so you can report *his* feelings, too.

When a problem's resolved
Draw a line through resolved or inactive problems with a yellow marker. In this way, you can tell at a glance which problems need attention, and which are discontinued. Remember, never use any marker that would completely cover what's been written; *a chart is a legal record.*

Knowing who does what

Now let's examine the final way a proper care plan helps: It serves as a guide for making patient care assignments. For example, if you're a team leader, you may want to delegate some of the specific routines or duties in each approach. Not all of them need your professional attention.

However, remember you can't delegate your professional *judgment* when you assign patient care; you can delegate only *duties*. Suppose, for instance, you're caring for a patient with hypertension. You may want to assign an aide to *take* his blood pressure, but you will have to make a judgment on the reading.

Keep monitoring your plan to make sure it's implemented correctly. If you don't — and part of your plan fails — you won't know whether it was the wrong approach to the problem, or just improper implementation.

How to write a care plan

Now that I've explained *why* care plans are written — and how they help — let's consider *how* they're written. You must observe certain rules when you prepare a care plan, or it'll lose some of its effectiveness.

To begin with, think of your care plan as the problem-solving part of the nursing process — which you learned about in Chapter 1. It's the plan of action you've chosen to solve the patient's problems, *after* you assessed his condition, identified his problems, established goals, and considered all alternative approaches or solutions.

Never call it a *nursing* care plan. Always refer to it as a *patient* care plan. You write it to elicit a positive response from your patient, so all orders in it must be written with that in mind.

Who's responsible for starting the patient's care plan? If you assessed and evaluated him initially, *you* are — although every nurse caring for that patient during his hospital stay must update it. So let's take this part of the nursing process step-by-step, so you know how to proceed.

Begin by identifying the patient's problems and listing them, as you learned to do in Chapter 6. Then consider the goals you want your patient to reach, as a result of your care.

Mutually agreeable goals: The long and short of it

What about those goals? Some authorities believe the goals for

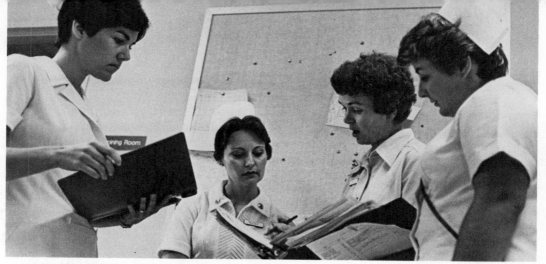

AVOIDING PROBLEMS WITH AN ADEQUATE CARE PLAN

A well-conceived and properly written care plan, besides doing other things, can spare your patient needless suffering. In writing your patients' care plans, try to anticipate *all* potential problems. Then, take measures to avoid them.

Here are several examples of problems that could have been avoided with an adequate care plan:

Case 1

Two days after 81-year-old Hannah Coleman was admitted to the hospital, the night shift nurse discovered her lying on the floor near her bed. The doctor was called immediately, and – after an X-ray examination – confirmed that Mrs. Coleman had a fractured pelvis. When he asked her why she'd climbed out of bed, Mrs. Coleman hesitated. "I thought I was home in my own bedroom," she said, confused, "...and I was looking for my cat."

Now, let's put you in this picture. With a good care plan, you might have prevented this unfortunate accident. How? First, recognize Mrs. Coleman's advanced age as a potential problem. An elderly patient who's just been admitted to the hospital can easily become confused at night in unfamiliar surroundings. To prevent an accident from occurring in a situation like this, write all or some of these precautions into the patient's care plan: (1) Put side rails up on bed. (2) Make half-hourly checks through the night. (3) Keep patient's night light on.

Case 2

Sixty-three-year-old Beatrice Quinn couldn't sleep the night before her cholecystectomy. Without considering all the possible causes for Mrs. Quinn's sleeplessness, the night shift attributed it to preop anxiety. However, Mrs. Quinn continued to have trouble sleeping after her surgery. When the nurse looked into the situation further, she learned that Mrs. Quinn's anxiety was caused by a problem at home. The previous year her husband had suffered a stroke, which had left him partially paralyzed. Also, the Quinns had lost their son and daughter-in-law in an accident and had the four grandchildren living with them.

Now let's put you in this picture. With a good care plan, you might have relieved some of Mrs. Quinn's anxiety and perhaps prevented her insomnia. How?

First, you'd examine all possible causes for Mrs. Quinn's sleeplessness the minute she complained of it. You'd ask her what *she* thought was causing it, as well as studying the information available on her initial assessment form. Then when you discovered that her home situation was the root of her anxiety, you'd include these instructions in her care plan: (1) Arrange for a home-health aide to care for the patient's husband and prepare meals for the family. (2) Call the children at 7:00 a.m. daily to wake them for school, or arrange for someone else to do it. (3) Get permission for the older grandchildren to visit the patient after school hours.

Case 3

Walter Philips, a 71-year-old retired accountant, was hospitalized for surgical removal of a cataract on his left eye. His vision in his right eye was functional, provided he wore corrective lenses. However, after surgery, Mr. Philips couldn't wear his glasses because of the patch and shield over his left eye. No one realized he was temporarily "blind" because of this, and Mr. Philips fell, injuring his arm.

Now let's put you in this picture. With a good care plan, you might have prevented this unfortunate accident. How?

First, anticipate that Mr. Philips will have a problem seeing without his glasses. Advise him of this, so he'll know you will care for him. Then identify the problem as a temporary one in your Kardex or problem list, and write the following instructions in his care plan: Assist patient with activities of daily living and help him to walk until he can wear his corrective lenses again.

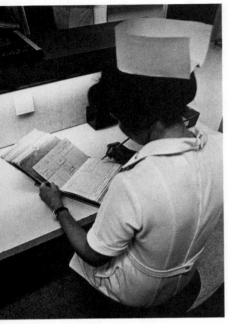

Keeping it current
Taking time to update your patients' Kardex care plans, like this nurse is doing, protects you and your patients from errors. Here's an example of what could happen if you didn't indicate resolved problems on your care plans:

After reading an unfamiliar patient's Kardex, a p.r.n. nurse approached him with gloves, dressings, and antibiotic ointment to care for his infected wound. Much to her chagrin, the patient's wound had long since healed. No one had taken the trouble to cross the resolved problem off his care plan.

the patient are the outcome criteria defined by the nursing audit committee. (This relationship can be seen in Chapter 12.)

However, other authorities feel that you should set the goals you want your patient to reach after you identify his problems. Along with each goal, you should also list a realistic target date for that goal to be reached. This immediately gives you two categories of goals — or expected outcomes — to consider: long- and short-term.

Some problems obviously can't be completely resolved before the patient's discharge: for example, a woman's adjustment to a radical mastectomy. So, you'll have to include these long-term problems in your discharge planning, and write your care plans accordingly.

When you set goals for your patient to achieve, remember to consider his thoughts about those goals, if he's physically and mentally able to give them to you. Perhaps he doesn't agree with your expected outcomes for his problems. Maybe he doesn't even understand them. Always talk to your patient about his problems before you write a care plan; begin doing this at the conclusion of your interview. Then set goals that are mutually agreeable, so you'll both be participating actively — and willingly — in the care plan.

Selecting your approach

Now, you're ready to study alternative approaches to your patient's problems. This, of course, takes time and effort. You must first review all the initial assessment data you've collected to see if you'll require further information. Then you must consider the patient's individual characteristics and needs, so you'll know which approach will work best for him.

Never standardize your approach to a specific problem. Always individualize it. Remember, no two problems are exactly the same; every patient is an individual.

You've now selected the approach — or plan of action — you want to try. How can you be sure it's the right one? Obviously no guarantee can accompany each approach — no matter how carefully you've formulated it. One of the reasons you set target dates for each problem to be solved is to evaluate the response you're getting with your approach. Then, if it's not working, you can use an alternative approach — or devise a completely new one.

Nursing tip: Before you make a final decision on the approach you want to use, check it against the goal you and your patient have set — and see if you've overlooked anything. Is your goal *specific* enough to formulate a correct approach? Perhaps you should rewrite the goal. If you've made it too general, you'll have trouble writing an approach that's specific.

How to write each approach

Now you're ready to write your approaches — or nursing orders — for each problem. Together, they form your patient care plan. (Remember, however, that the patient's *total* care plan is the sum of everything that's done for him by the entire health-care team.)

Always write your care plan *in ink* (and sign it), even though you may have to revise it if your approaches don't work. Your patient's care plan becomes part of his *permanent* record, and should not be erased or destroyed. If you write it in pencil — so you can erase to revise — you make it seem unimportant. Care plans must remain intact, enabling you and other health-team members to readily refer to approaches used in the past.

Consider these things when you write your care plan:
- what observations to make and how often
- what nursing measures to take and how to implement them
- what to teach the patient and/or his family before he's discharged.

The first phase refers to the ongoing assessment process that you always include in the care of every patient. Your orders should specify what to *observe,* what to *inspect,* and what to learn through an *interview*.

For example, let's suppose you're caring for a patient who had a cerebrovascular accident. And one of the problems requiring management on his list is urinary incontinence. You might write the first phase of your approach as follows:

Date	D/C'd date	Problem	Goal	Target date	Approach (nursing order)
10/14		CVA — urinary incontinence	Remain free of urinary tract infection or receive prompt treatment for urinary tract infection	Duration of catheter insertion	Be alert for signs of urinary tract infection, temperature above 100° and cloudy, foul-smelling urine, with or without pain and burning.

Now, let's consider the second phase of patient care to include in your approach: What nursing measures to do and how to do them. Make these very specific, so there's no confusion about what to do. For your patient with urinary incontinence, you might add to your orders like this:

Date	D/C'd date	Problem	Goal	Target date	Approach (nursing order)
Same		Same	Same	Same	Catheter care routine (see Procedure Manual) at beginning of each shift. Change catheter tubing and drainage bag if sediment accumulates or in 14 days — tape date on bag. Ensure adequate oral fluid intake 1420 cc (7-3 shift) 1100 cc (3-11 shift) 480 cc (11-7 shift).

The third phase of patient care to include in your approach involves patient/family education. You must list what the patient and his family should be told or taught before discharge — and describe it specifically.

In the case of the patient we've been following, you might write these orders in your approach:

Date	D/C'd date	Problem	Goal	Target date	Approach (nursing order)
Same		Same	Same	by 10/15	Arrange for conference with wife to determine teaching schedule and target dates. RN to teach wife symptoms of urinary tract infection. RN to teach wife to irrigate Foley catheter using sterile technique. RN to review with wife printed instructions on care of catheter and drainage bag. RN to check return demonstrations on catheter care and irrigation. *E. Vasey, RN*

Be specific
As you can see from the completed sample on page 103

you must make your orders specific. Otherwise, your patient's care will lack continuity and the results will be unpredictable.

Suppose you *don't* make your orders specific. Each nurse might then rely on her own interpretation of what should be done. Or worse, she'll rely on the patient for instructions about his own care.

Be specific about times and dates in your orders. For example, suppose a patient with severe gastrointestinal pain is scheduled for a GI series on April 20, 3 days from the time you write your order. On the care plan, in the appropriate column, you'd write:

Date	D/C'd date	Problem	Goal	Target date	Approach (nursing order)
4/17		Lacks knowledge of GI series	Verbalize instructions on GI series	4/19 a.m.	RN to instruct patient on GI series preparation and and procedure. *E. Vasey, RN*

The creative approach
Try to be creative in your approach to a patient's problem. Draw a sketch of what you mean, if it'll help. For example, suppose a patient with a fractured hip needs pillows placed about him in a certain way: Illustrate it with a drawing on your care plan.

Here's another creative approach successfully used in a care plan for a patient with Guillain-Barre syndrome. Because of her illness, she had great difficulty communicating. But she could wiggle her toes, so an innovative nurse devised a way for her to answer questions with them. She instructed the patient to wiggle her right toe for "yes" and her left toe for "no." Then she documented this entire approach on the patient's care plan, so each nurse caring for her had a way to communicate.

Don't forget anything
Try hard not to forget any of your patient's needs or concerns when you write his care plan. Check over your initial assessment data thoroughly. Never rely on word-of-mouth to care for a patient's needs. Write all specific instructions that relate to a patient's problems, needs, or concerns on the care plan.

For example, I heard about a woman patient who specifi-

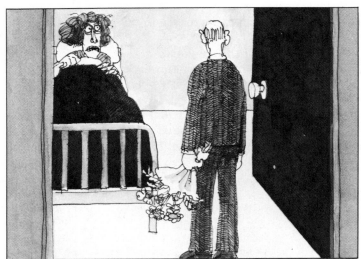

cally told the nurse doing her assessment that she didn't want her husband to visit her. The nurse recorded the information on the assessment sheet, but forgot to list it on the care plan. As a result, no one on the next shift knew about the woman's request. Her husband was allowed to visit her. And she became so hysterical that she needed medication ordered to sedate her.

Revising the plan

Now you know how to write your patient's care plan. Make sure it's implemented correctly by reviewing the documentation and assessing the patient. Then evaluate the results of your care plan to see if your goals have been accomplished.

If your approach has solved the patient's problem, write "discontinued" next to it on the care plan, and list the date you discontinued that approach. If your approach hasn't solved the patient's problem by the target date, reevaluate it and do one of the following:

• Extend the target date and continue the approach until your patient responds as expected.

• Discontinue the approach and select a new one that will achieve the expected outcome.

In the next chapter, you'll learn more about why some care plans fail. Before you go on to Chapter 8, review what you've learned here about how to write a care plan.

PATIENT CARE PLAN

Date	D/C'd date	Problem	Goal	Target date	Approach (nursing order)
10/14		CVA — urinary incontinence	Remain free of urinary tract infection or receive prompt treatment for urinary tract infection	Duration of catheter insertion	Be alert for signs of urinary tract infection, temperature above 100° and cloudy, foul-smelling urine, with or without pain and burning. Catheter care routine (see Procedure Manual) at beginning of each shift. Change catheter tubing and drainage bag if sediment accumulates or in 14 days — tape date on bag. Ensure adequate oral fluid intake 1420 cc (7-3 shift) 1100 cc (3-11 shift) 480 cc (11-7 shift).
				by 10/15	Arrange for conference with wife to determine teaching schedule and target dates. RN to teach wife symptoms of urinary tract infection. RN to teach wife to irrigate Foley catheter using sterile technique. RN to review with wife printed instructions on care of catheter and drainage bag. RN to check return demonstrations on catheter care and irrigation.

E. Vasey, RN

Remember these rules about how to write a care plan:

1. Always write your patient's care plans in ink. They are a part of his permanent record. Sign your name.
2. Take time to review all your assessment data *before* you select an approach for each problem.
3. Write down a specific goal — or expected outcome — for each problem on the list, and record a target date for its completion.
4. Write an approach or nursing order for each problem on the list.
5. Consider the following three phases of patient care in every approach you write: What observations to make and how often; what nursing measures to do and how to do them; what to teach the patient and his family before discharge.
6. Make each nursing order or approach specific.
7. Be creative when you write your patient's care plan; include a drawing or innovative procedure, if either will make the order more specific.
8. Don't overlook any of the patient's problems or concerns. Include them on the care plan, so they won't be forgotten.
9. Make sure your care plan is implemented correctly.
10. Evaluate the results of your care plan and discontinue those problems that have been resolved. Select new approaches, if necessary, for problems that have not been resolved.

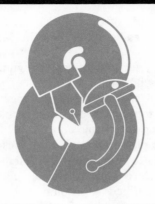

PLANNING PATIENT CARE
Why some care plans fail

BY IRENE M. LEE, RN, BA

HAVE YOU EVER READ a care plan like this?

Date	D/C'd date	Problem	Goal	Target date	Approach (nursing orders)
5/10		Dehydration	Exhibit no symptoms of fluid depletion		Force fluids

Then you've seen why some care plans fail. They're so filled with vague generalities that they're meaningless in directing patient care.

But care plans fail to accomplish set goals for other reasons. Do you know what those reasons are? If you're at all uncertain, you need to read this chapter.

Pinpointing the cause
As you recall from reading Chapter 7, a well-conceived and properly written care plan helps you by:
- giving direction to patient care
- establishing continuity of care

Creative approach 1:
A nurse in Oregon reports that she helped a tracheostomy patient to communicate by using a child's magnetic letterboard. Although too weak to write, the patient could easily see the large letters and move them without much effort. With a few words, she could indicate her needs and desires to the health team. Furthermore, the activity helped stimulate her physically and mentally during her long illness.

You can adapt this technique for other speech-impaired patients, or for patients on respirators. And because this method takes less motor coordination than writing, it can also help patients with neurological disorders such as multiple sclerosis.

• providing a means of communication between you and other health-team professionals, and between you and the patient

• serving as a key for patient-care assignments.

Your care plan will fail if it doesn't meet any or all of these general goals. It will also fail if it doesn't meet the *specific* goal you've set for it: solving the patient's problems.

What goes wrong with some care plans? Based on experience, I'd say care plans fail mostly for these reasons:

• insufficient data to complete the problem-solving process

• one or more of the patient's physical, mental, or emotional deficits weren't identified as problems

• the approach chosen to solve a difficult or unusual problem wasn't innovative enough

• the plan was not specific.

The insufficient data base: Why it happens

Let's discuss the first reason care plans fail: the insufficient data base. As you learned earlier in this book, you can't accurately identify your patient's problems and work out his care plan without a complete initial assessment.

To collect the information you need, you must first interview, observe, and inspect the patient. To do this properly, use the techniques described in Chapters 3 and 4, and relate the information you collect to the patient's chief complaint.

If your patient can't be interviewed because of his condition, you may have to interview his family. Or you may have to talk to the persons accompanying him to the hospital: for example, the ambulance attendants.

Now, what can happen to keep you from collecting the data you need on a patient? Well, he may be admitted to the hospital too late at night for a complete assessment. If this happens, immediately identify "insufficient data base" as one of the patient's problems, and *document it*. Then the health-team professionals who care for him on the next shift will be alerted and gather the needed information before his care plan is written.

Learn to talk to your patient

You can fail to collect sufficient data for other reasons, however. And these shortcomings may be harder to discover. For example, you may lack the interviewing skills you need to get pertinent information — and simply not realize it.

Review what you learned in Chapter 3. Do you regularly use the important interviewing techniques described there? Or are you like some nurses I've met — so busy *doing* things for patients that they never really *talk* to them.

Suppose you realize you have difficulty interviewing patients. Analyze your problem. Perhaps you just lack experience and need to practice your skills repeatedly.

No time?

If you say you lack the *time* to interview your patients properly, you're citing a difficulty that plagues most of us. My advice is to *use* what time you have more effectively. Make every encounter you have with each patient a *meaningful one*.

Let me illustrate exactly what I'm talking about here. How many times a shift do you enter a patient's room? And what do you say to that patient when you're in there? I've actually seen some nurses say *nothing* — or some say something vague like, "How are you?" They throw away the opportunity they have to communicate with that patient, and thus fail to collect what might have been valuable data.

What are you *really* saying?

Check out the nonverbal messages you convey to your patient. They may be keeping you from getting the information you need from him. For example, do you avoid eye contact? Are you always in a hurry? Is your voice crisp and formal?

If you constantly give the impression that you really don't want to know how he's feeling, he probably won't tell you. Once again, you'll have missed an opportunity to keep your data base up to date.

Avoid meaningless chitchat when you talk to your patient. For example, don't waste time discussing the weather. Use that valuable time to explain the therapy or tests he'll have that day. Or teach him more about his condition or illness. Is it apt to affect his life-style — or his family's — when he's discharged? Encourage him to tell you how. He may have fears and worries he wants to discuss, but won't mention them unless you ask.

Missed any important clues, lately?

But lack of practice at interviewing isn't the only reason you

Creative approach 2
Mabel Hoskins was a 54-year-old cancer patient whose tumor had broken through the skin. Naturally, she was upset and embarrassed by its unpleasant odor and profuse drainage. Because of this, she refused to leave her room or accept visitors. This self-imposed quarantine seriously affected Mrs. Hoskins. Her emotional resources were quickly exhausted, and she began sinking into a profound depression.

Accurately assessing the cause of Mrs. Hoskins' depression, the nurse applied a dressing over the ulcerated area, then covered it with a denture cup, minimizing the odor. Overnight, Mrs. Hoskins' spirits improved. She began taking walks in the hall once again and greeted her visitors warmly.

Nursing tip: Determine the *real* cause of a patient's problem. Once you understand it clearly, you can look for a way to solve it that's both practical and creative.

Creative approach 3
After 18 days in a ventilator, 70-year-old Anna Tyler began to feel cut off from reality. "Time just drifts by. I don't even know what day of the week this is," she confessed anxiously to her nurse. Remembering that Ms. Tyler had indeed been asking the time and date with increasing frequency, the nurse began to devise a plan to help combat her disorientation.

To the inside of the ventilator, Ms. Tyler's nurse taped a chart naming the days of the week, with each day represented by a different color. Then, each morning she pinned a strip of appropriately colored cloth to the front of Ms. Tyler's gown.

The nurse's plan worked. Ms. Tyler was now able to tell at a glance what day it was, and once more felt in touch with the world.

may fail to get a complete data base. You may be missing important clues when you observe and inspect your patient.

Do you always know exactly what data to look for when a patient has a specific complaint? Do you collect them systematically? If you think you can improve on your skills in this area, review Chapter 4.

Determining the deficits

What's another big reason care plans fail? You may have missed one of the patient's problems. Remember, you must look on any physical, mental, or emotional deficit as a problem, if it may interfere with his care or well-being. Some authorities call these coping deficits, and label them by categories. For example, a patient may have one or more deficits in these areas:

- strength
- endurance
- sensory input
- knowledge
- desire
- courage
- skill dexterity
- support systems.

Let me give you several examples of what I mean by this. Suppose your patient has a deficit in knowledge. Many patients do, of course, which is why you must do so much patient teaching.

A patient about to have abdominal surgery may have no idea of what to expect. His lack of knowledge may interfere with his care plan, unless you recognize his deficit and take steps to correct it.

Don't just teach your patient the "usual" things when you prepare him for surgery: for instance, coughing, turning, deep-breathing. Try to imagine some of the misconceptions he may have. Any of them could affect his care in the hospital — and possibly cause serious difficulties. For example, an uninformed patient may:

- assume that you'll automatically give him his pain medication when he needs it, without his request
- fear that his pain medication will turn him into a drug addict
- fear that the sutures in his incision will pop open if he coughs and moves, as instructed

- assume that his condition is deteriorating because of frequent vital signs checks.

Since he won't realize these are only misconceptions, he may not ask about them. You'll just have to imagine what each patient may be thinking — based on your experience, your intuition, and your assessment of the patient's education level.

Relieving fears about the unknown

Remember to explain all scheduled diagnostic tests to your patient. He may have only a vague idea about what's going to happen to him during testing. In some cases, the distorted reality of television and movies may have magnified his fears to unrealistic proportions.

For example, while I was checking on an elderly woman patient of mine one day, I was dismayed to find her crying. When I asked what was wrong, she tearfully replied that she was afraid to have a scheduled scanning test. I quickly explained how this test was given, and her relief was instantaneous. "You can't imagine how much sleep I've lost over this" she cried, hugging me. "I thought an isotope was like an electric shock."

Your responsibility to know

Are you thinking, "I don't know what happens during every diagnostic test." Well, I say it's your responsibility to know. How can you help your patient to overcome his knowledge deficits in this area if you don't know much about it yourself?

Actually, several ways exist for you to keep abreast the latest diagnostic procedures. For example, you can learn more about them through an intradepartmental inservice program. Or you can observe many of the procedures directly by visiting the department. Or you can read up on them.

Sensory deficits: Another problem

Now let's suppose your patient has a sensory deficit. That can also affect his care plan. For example, imagine you have a surgical patient who is almost blind. How can you write a care plan that will fulfill his needs? If you write a plan that's suited to a sighted surgical patient, your blind patient will suffer. Obviously, you must consider his sensory deficit as a problem and write a care plan that deals with it.

For example, you might plan to arrange his meal trays in a

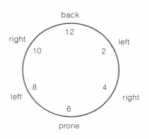

(a.m. and p.m.)

Open to question

"Give an antihypertensive drug by a convenient route, several times this week." If you ever saw a doctor's order like that, you'd question it immediately, and rightly so. The order doesn't tell you anything specific about the drug, the time, or the dosage, or the route of administration.

Now suppose a patient's care plan contained the following *nursing* order: "Implement effective measures to prevent skin breakdown." Would you question it? You should! Like doctors' orders, a nursing order isn't properly written unless it's specific and detailed. In this case, it should say something like: "Turn patient every 2 hours (on even hours), according to diagram."

consistent pattern, so he can easily remember where each food item is located. Then draw a rough sketch of this pattern on your written care plan, so every nurse can follow it.

Problem	Approach (nursing orders)
¾ totally blind — will be able to feed self with minimum assistance	At each meal, arrange tray in the following way: 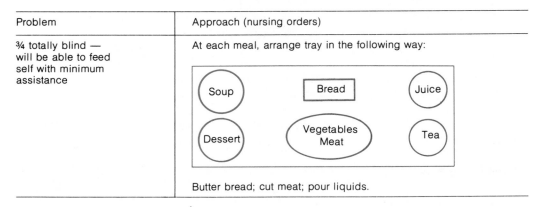 Butter bread; cut meat; pour liquids.

Difficult problem? Try an innovative approach

What's another reason your care plan could fail? Perhaps the approach chosen to solve the patient's problem wasn't innovative enough. Obviously, you need to spend time — and stretch your imagination — to come up with workable strategies.

In Chapter 7, you learned about a creative approach used for a patient with Guillian-Barre syndrome, and on the previous pages you learned some others. Draw the inspiration you need from these examples, and be as innovative as you can when you're faced with difficult problems in your patients.

Getting the patient ready to go home

Keep in mind that any coping deficit can affect more than your care plans for him while he's in the hospital. It can affect your plans for him when he returns home and has to care for himself.

For example, if he lacks support from his family during his recovery, he may be too discouraged to complete the self-care procedures you've outlined for him. Or he may lack the knowledge he needs to fully understand how to care for himself, as you'll learn later in Chapter 11.

Be specific

Now, here's the last reason why care plans fail: You aren't specific enough when you write your nursing orders. For example, I've seen care plans like the one at the beginning of this chapter and realized how meaningless they are.

Now here's another one, written for a patient suffering from side effects of chemotherapy. See how nonspecific it is in its present form, then learn how to improve it.

Date	D/C'd date	Problem	Goal	Target date	Approach (nursing orders)
3/4/78		4 Weight loss from nausea and vomiting	Restore to optimum state of health		Encourage oral intake

Now, let's write a care plan that's specific enough for a patient with the same problem — and outline everything you want done. Notice how the nursing orders differ in these two examples, and how much easier it would be to follow the orders in the example below.

Date	D/C'd date	Problem	Goal	Target date	Approach (nursing orders)
3/4/78		4 Potential weight loss from nausea and vomiting	4 a. Maintains the admission weight b. Takes most of all meals without nausea or vomiting c. Verbalizes understand-ing of diet	Disch Vq8h	4 a. Weigh daily at 7:30 a.m. be-fore breakfast b. Offer high protein, high calorie drinks between meals c. Offer meals in 6 small feedings d. Give antiemetic at 8 a.m., 12 noon, 4 p.m., and 8 p.m. e. Have dietician explain diet and find about food preferences f. Encourage family to bring favorite foods from home

What are some other things to remember about being specific? Write in a way that everyone will understand. For example, avoid using vague terms like "provide adequate rest," "force fluids," and "give emotional support."

Instead, say exactly how many hours of rest you expect the patient to have — and at what time; and how many milliliters of fluid you want him to take at various times throughout the day. Don't say, "Give emotional support"; say how much time each shift of nurses should spend at the patient's bedside to accomplish this.

Don't use abbreviations that can be confused with ones meaning something quite different. First, check out our lengthy list of commonly confused medical and nursing abbreviations in the appendix of this book. Then make sure everyone you work with uses the same ones.

All these precautions add up to make effective care plans that are easy to follow. And that's all you expect from any care plan — and all you need to insure quality care.

Don't let your patient care plans fail because you've overlooked one or more of the important points I've outlined in this chapter. Keep them in mind, as you go on to read the rest of this book.

Remember these rules for writing successful care plans:

1. **If you can't complete the initial patient assessment, immediately identify "insufficient data base" as a problem.**
2. **If you can't interview your patient due to his condition, collect data from his family or persons accompanying him to the hospital.**
3. **If you have difficulty getting the information you need in an interview, check out the nonverbal messages you convey to your patient to see if they're negative.**
4. **Use your interview time effectively; make every encounter with your patient a meaningful one.**
5. **Before you observe and inspect your patient, review the doctor's admitting diagnosis. This will keep you from overlooking important clues related to the patient's condition.**
6. **Include physical, mental, or emotional deficits as problems if they could interfere with your patient's care or well-being.**
7. **Try to imagine some of the misconceptions your patient may have and take steps to correct them.**
8. **Spend time and stretch your imagination to devise innovative approaches to your patient's problems.**
9. **Be specific; don't use vague terms or generalities on the care plan.**
10. **Never use abbreviations that may be confused with ones meaning something quite different.**

SKILLCHECK 3

1. The latest entry has just been made on Margaret O'Toole's problem list:

Date onset	No.	Active problems (acute and chronic)	Name	Date resolved	Inactive or resolved problems
4/3/78	1	4/5/78 GI bleeding, peptic ulcer	M. Jones, RN		
	2		M. Jones, RN	1965	Thyroidectomy
1956	3	Diabetes	M. Jones, RN		
4/3/78	4	Skin rash	M. Jones, RN	4/7/78	
4/4/78	5	Concern over absence from job	M. Jones, RN	4/8/78	

Which of these conclusions is justified?
a) Margaret currently has 5 active problems.
b) Peptic ulcer and diabetes are the only active problems Margaret has.
c) GI bleeding and skin rash shouldn't have been identified on the active problem list.
d) Thyroidectomy should be identified as an active chronic problem even if there are no residual effects.

2. Read the following excerpt from a patient care plan:

Date	D/C'd date	Problem	Goal	Target date	Approach (nursing order)
9/12		Need for post-operative instructions	Patient demonstrates deep breathing, coughing, turning and exercises	Day before surgery	Teach deep breathing, coughing, turning and exercises

Which of these answers is an accurate critique?
a) The approach is not innovative enough.
b) The problem is not related to the approach.
c) The goal is not measurable.
d) The approach is not specific.

3. You are the only RN on the evening shift and six patients have been admitted to your care. Your initial patient assessments have focused on priorities only. What is your next step?
a) Tell the RN on the night shift to complete the assessments.
b) Immediately identify "insufficient data base" as a problem on the problem list and/or care plan.
c) Place only the urgent problems on the problem list and/or Kardex care plan.
d) Delegate the responsibility for completing the assessments to the nursing aide.

4. Andrew Smolsky, 84, was admitted with a diagnosis of possible cancer of the urinary bladder. Ten years ago he had pyelonephritis, which has been resolved. His chief complaint now is hematuria. You've just overheard the doctors discussing a possible transurethral resection. Which of the following problems would be entered under the Active Problems column on the problem list?
a) Hematuria
b) Pyelonephritis
c) Cancer of the urinary bladder
d) Transurethral resection of prostate gland.

5. You notice that many of your patients seem ill at ease when you interview them, and reluctant to communicate with you. Which step do you take next to correct this situation?
a) Request that interviewing be done by another nurse.
b) Insist that your patients communicate more effectively to improve care.
c) Determine if you're conveying any negative nonverbal messages that cause your patients' behavior.
d) Let interviews go for several days until the patients are more comfortable.

(Answers on page 180)

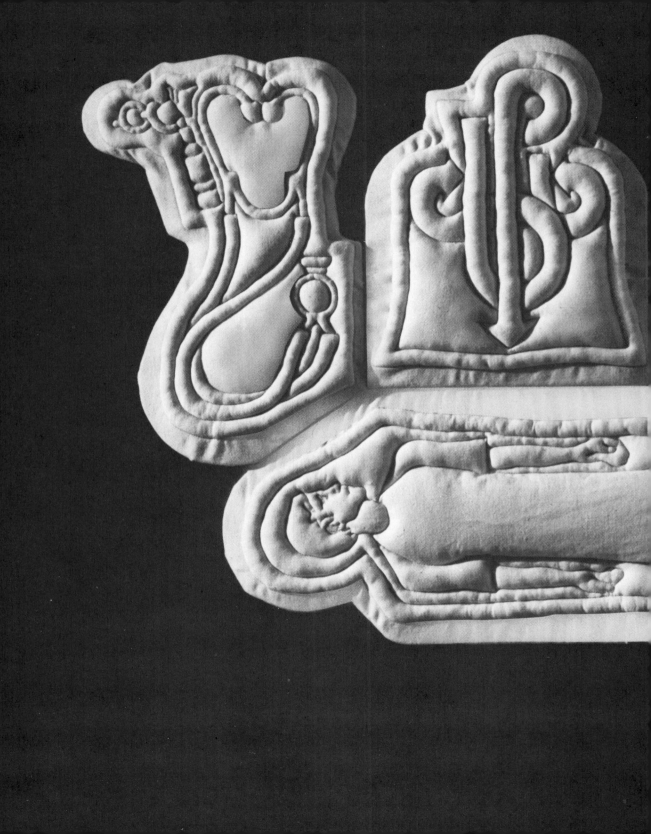

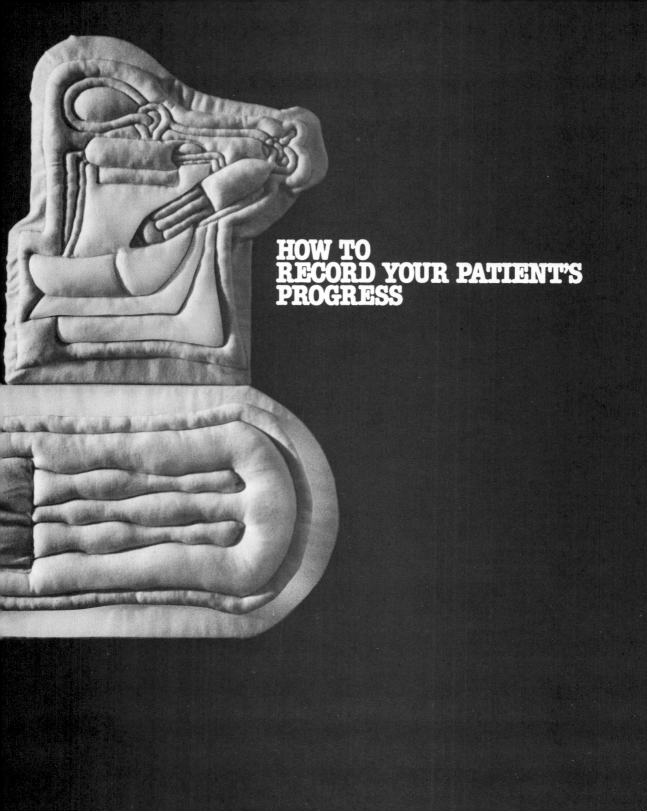

HOW TO
RECORD YOUR PATIENT'S
PROGRESS

"When you chart a patient's progress,
don't just collect
meaningless data and document it.
Record only significant findings."

"Always document
your patient's response
to his care.
It's the only way you can properly
evaluate his care plan
and determine if it's effective."

"Think of your notes as a camera
that takes the patient's picture.
Be so specific
that anyone who reads your notes
will be able to see
that patient through your words."

"Start planning for your patient's
discharge from the day of his admission.
Then before you write his discharge summary,
review his care plan and
initial assessment form."

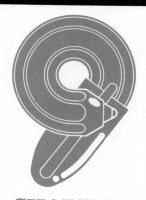

CHARTING YOUR PATIENT'S PROGRESS
How to use the problem-oriented system

BY MARY M. REILLY, RN, BSN

WHAT SORT OF PROGRESS NOTES do you see in *your* unit? Entries like this one, which was written about a patient about to have an emergency appendectomy?

Date	Time	Progress notes
12/16/77	4 PM	Pt. c/o abdominal pain. I.V. running OK. Shaving prep for O.R. Gave routine preop teaching.
	5 PM	To O.R. M. Reilly, RN

If notes like this look familiar, then you're aware how little they communicate when they're poorly written — and how confusing they can be, as a result.

For example, how much does the above note actually tell you about the patient? How does she feel about having emergency surgery? Is she frightened? Was she given any *medication* to sedate her before surgery? And what was her *response* to it? What exactly did the nurse explain during the routine preop teaching session? How much did the patient understand?

Incognito
Meet a mystery patient.
According to the most recent entry
on his chart, he's in for X-ray for a
GI series — and at the same time
is receiving an I.V. of 5% dextrose
in water at 100 ml/hr. Everything
else about him is left to your
imagination, as you can see from
this picture. You don't know what
his chief complaint is, if he has
any other symptoms, or if he was
taught anything about the tests
he's having.

Nursing tip: Keep in mind that
your notes serve as a camera.
Write enough to take a complete
picture of your patient, so others
know all they should about him.

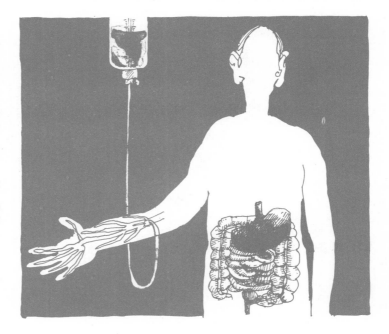

The unstructured paragraph

Obviously, you can't learn much about the patient from a
progress note like this. Not only is it vague, but everything
about the patient and her problems is lumped haphazardly into
one paragraph. So I'm going to take this same patient and
show you how her progress notes should look. You'll be
reading about her in the next three chapters, because I'll be
discussing her case right up to the point when she's discharged.

As you know, the note I've just illustrated is written in a
narrative paragraph style, which is characteristic of source-
oriented progress notes. In source-oriented notes, no structured format exists to help you organize and relate your
documentation to the patient's problems. Furthermore, the
system offers no built-in guide to show you what's important
to document. So you may find yourself grouping everything
together in long, disorganized paragraphs. Instead of talking
about one problem per paragraph, you may discuss three or
four.

But wait. Am I saying that source-oriented progress notes
must always be poorly written? Of course not. Many of you

use the source-oriented system in your hospital and do very well with it. However, for those of you who still have trouble writing meaningful notes within this system, I suggest reading Chapter 10. In that chapter, I'll discuss your particular difficulties at length — and explain how to improve your documentation, no matter which system (or combination of systems) you use.

Introducing the POMR progress note

But now, I want to tell you about problem-oriented progress notes, which are preferred by many hospitals because they're more structured. Built into the notes is a specific format, which you already know corresponds to the letters SOAPIER.

Before I explain what these letters stand for, let me tell you still another way POMR progress notes differ from the source-oriented system. In POMR notes, you no longer write all the information you want to record about your patient's problems in one long paragraph. You write separate SOAP entries for each problem you've identified on the patient's problem list.

Think back to Chapters 6 and 7. That's where you learned how to write the formal problem list your patient will need for his POMR progress notes. It's also where you learned to write an initial care plan that corresponds to the numbered problems on the list. You see, each SOAP entry you write must have *more* than the date and time next to it; it must also have the *name and number of the problem it relates to*. Then your documentation stays organized, and you can quickly review a problem's course by referring back to its number.

Getting to know Mary Anthony

You'll see how easy this works when we discuss the case of Mary Anthony. She's the patient I talked about earlier in this chapter — the one who came in for an emergency appendectomy. Before I say any more about her, read pages 182 through 185 in the appendix. That's where you'll find Ms. Anthony's completed assessment form, her problem list, and her initial care plan.

As you can see from the initial assessment form, Ms. Anthony is a 45-year-old vocalist in a supper club. And shortly after rehearsal one morning, she went to her doctor complaining of severe pain in her right lower quadrant. He immediately

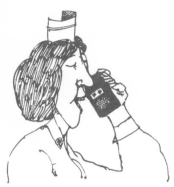

No time to chart?
Finding time to keep up with patient charting isn't as easy as it sounds. For example, what do you do on a night when you're the only RN on a 32-bed unit and you have: two new admissions; a disoriented patient who's already broken three Posey restraints; a recent postop patient whose urine output is decreasing steadily; three patients who are complaining they can't sleep; and a 320-lb stroke patient who needs turning every two hours?

Temporarily record the most important details about each patient you care for in a pocket tape recorder. Then later that night, write your complete notes on the patient's permanent record.

Important: Whenever you tape record notes, always identify each patient you're discussing, the time and date, and yourself. Then to protect yourself, in case the entry is questioned, keep the tape for several days after you've transcribed it.

Here's a shopping tip: All miniature tape recorders have built-in mikes and sell for less than $100. Most of them accept standard compact size cassettes. Others, however, are designed to accept only the manufacturer's special cassettes. Check before you buy.

suspected appendicitis upon examining her, and had her admitted to a nearby hospital. There, she had all the laboratory tests needed to confirm the diagnosis, plus a complete assessment.

Now, let's imagine you work in that same hospital — in fact, in the same unit. And when you report for duty at 3 p.m., you find that Ms. Anthony is one of your patients. By the time you see her at 3:30 p.m., you know that her diagnosis of appendicitis has already been confirmed. Ms. Anthony is scheduled for an appendectomy at 5:30 p.m.

Since your hospital uses the POMR system, you can refer to more than Ms. Anthony's updated assessment form and Kardex before you begin her care. You can also review her problem list and initial plan, both of which have been updated — like the assessment form — to include her confirmed diagnosis (see pages 183 and 184).

Then you can start preparing her for surgery, as indicated in the care plan. This plan is very specific, as you can see, so you know exactly what you're expected to do about each numbered problem — as well as what to document.

How to write the SOAPIER note
Now you've come to the part where you write your first POMR progress note about Ms. Anthony — using the SOAPIER format. And you'll write it about her number one problem: appendicitis. So it's time to explain what each SOAPIER letter means, in the order you'll record it. *Remember, each problem gets its own SOAPIER data. You never include more than one problem in each SOAPIER entry.*

Now here's the format:

• S: Subjective data (the patient's symptoms, or what she tells you she feels)

• O: Objective data (the patient's signs, or the factual data you gather by observing and inspecting her)

• A: Assessment (the conclusion you come to about your patient's problem)

• P: Plan of care (what you plan to do about your patient's problem now or in the future)

• I: Intervention (what you've already done to, for, or with her, relative to this problem)

• E: Evaluation (the outcome of your intervention; was it effective or ineffective?)

• R: Revision (how you've changed the care plan, if your intervention hasn't proved successful).

Subjective data

Now that you have some idea what SOAPIER notes are all about, let's go back to the first thing you'll record on your entry about Ms. Anthony. This is your S data, where you consider her feelings or reactions to a particular problem. For example, you'd write what your patient tells you she feels — as a direct quote or in a summarization. In Ms. Anthony's case, she says she feels a "little nervous, and will be glad when her surgery is over."

Date	Time	No.	Problem	Patient progress notes
12/16/77	4 PM	1	Appendicitis	S: "A little nervous; will be glad when surgery is over."

Remember, since the letter S refers to the patient's subjective experience, you needn't write "the patient states..." You already have made this understood by listing the information under the letter S.

However, if the patient is unable to give you subjective data, you may have to ask his family for it. In that case, always document who gave you the information. Write something like "Ms. Anthony's brother states she is feeling a little nervous about her upcoming surgery."

What do you do if you have no S data to relate? Suppose, for example, your patient was unconscious and couldn't answer any questions. Just write the letter S after your entry and list the reason why you were unable to get the information. Then other health-team professionals who read your note will know that you haven't just ignored the S category.

Objective data

Now, let's consider the O part of your entry — the objective data. This is factual data that you've collected when you've observed or inspected your patient. Your senses provide you with the tools necessary to collect O data. You can also get O data from taking the patient's vital signs, or from laboratory tests and X-rays.

In Ms. Anthony's case, you'll record this data, as follows:

Date	Time	No.	Problem	Patient progress notes
				O: T. 99⁸ P. 88 R 18 BP 124/78; I.V. infusing in ® antecubital space. Operative area has been prepped.

Notice that your entry didn't mention that 5% dextrose in water (100 ml/hr) was being infused through the I.V. That's because such data is recorded on the doctor's orders and the patient's flow sheet. Duplication of data isn't necessary on the progress notes. Usually, you'll find it enough just to summarize the data.

In most cases, you won't even list the patient's vital signs in your O entry. You do that only when you want to call attention to them or, in this case, if it's your first encounter with a patient scheduled for surgery. Usually, you record vital signs on the patient's flow sheet — the proper place for documenting repetitive tasks. (Flow sheets serve many functions in both POMR and source-oriented systems. I'll tell you more about them later.)

What are some other examples of O data? Remember, O data is anything you can observe by using physical assessment techniques. For instance, you may record any of these findings: purulent drainage, dyspnea, patient crying, clammy skin, 1000 ml urine, slurred speech, or white blood cell count (WBC) 16,000.

Always focus your attention in the areas that will yield the most information about the patient's chief complaint. Don't just collect meaningless data and document it. Record only significant findings.

Assessment data
Next to the A in your entry, record the conclusions you've

come to about your S and O data; in other words, your *assessment* of your previous findings (S + O = A).

Your A data always indicates what's going on with your patient, and can show either progression, regression, or no change in her condition. *You may even state you don't know what's going on, because sometimes you won't be sure.*

However, never repeat a confirmed diagnosis when you document your A data, because this is not the place for it. Instead, write how the patient's disease or condition is progressing or regressing. And if no change exists in the patient's condition, simply write "no change."

You can see how to do this in Ms. Anthony's case. Next to A, write the following:

Date	Time	No.	Problem	Patient progress notes
				A: Expected preop apprehension

Later, when she returns from surgery, you'll have more to say in your A data — but that'll be in another entry. In fact, if you look ahead on Ms. Anthony's completed POMR progress notes on pages 126 and 127, you can see some of that data now.

Now, here are some other examples of A data that will help you understand what goes into this category: "skin breakdown secondary to immobilization"; "skin rash and itchiness secondary to medication"; "condition deteriorating rapidly over past 24 hours"; "disease controlled with medication and diet"; and "uncertain at this time as to cause of pain."

P for plan
In this part of your SOAPIER entry, you document what you plan to do about your patient's problem, now or in the future. And, of course, you base this on your most recent assessment — the A data in that particular entry. You also base it on the following guidelines:
- What additional information do you need to collect?
- What are you expected to do for the patient?
- What will you tell or teach him?

Let's take a look at what you'll record for Ms. Anthony under P data:

Date	Time	No.	Problem	Patient progress notes
				P: Will follow routine preop orders and preop teaching plan

Obviously, your S and O assessment data gives you no reason to question the plan outlined for Ms. Anthony. So you indicate that you'll complete the routine preop orders and teaching plan that are part of the initial plan.

However, if your S and O assessment data had suggested that another plan was needed to give your patient optimum care, you'd talk it over with your supervisor. But first, document what you think, and why, as well as the fact that you reported it.

I for implementation

Next to the letter I in your entry, write exactly what you've done to, for, or with your patient, about her problem. In other words, document your intervention — as illustrated here in your case about Ms. Anthony.

Date	Time	No.	Problem	Patient progress notes
				I: Recovery room explained. Coughing, turning, deep breathing and leg exercises explained and demonstrated. Pt. told that pain medication will be available postop, and to request it at onset of pain. Medicated and prepared for surgery.

Note how specific this entry is, and how much more it tells you than the sample entry at the very beginning of this chapter. This is the way an I entry should look; *it must never leave what you've done up to the reader's imagination.*

E for evaluation

Now let's consider the E part of your SOAPIER entry — the evaluation. Here's where you document your patient's *response* to your intervention, either positive or negative. For example, in Ms. Anthony's case, you write the following:

Date	Time	No.	Problem	Patient progress notes
				E: understands cough, turn, deep breathing and leg exercises — successfully returned demonstration. Med. effective — pt. drowsy. Relaxed on departure for O.R. M. Reilly, RN

R for revision

Ms. Anthony responds positively to your preop care. But sometimes a patient's response is not what you expect, and then you — or other health-team professionals — may have to revise care plans.

For example, suppose Ms. Anthony's preop medication wasn't effective within the specified time. You'd call the doctor immediately. Then you'd document his revised plan for medication next to the R in your entry.

SOAP or SOAPIER

Now take a look at the entire entry you've made for Ms. Anthony. You'll find it on page 126. On the same page, you'll find other SOAP and SOAPIER notes that were written about her for a short time postoperatively. As you can see, these include mention of another one of her problems — diabetes mellitus — which was listed on her assessment form, problem

PATIENT PROGRESS NOTES

NAME _Mary Anthony_

AGE _45_

DATE	TIME	NO.	PROBLEM	
12/16/77	4 PM	1	Appendicitis	S: "A little nervous. Will be glad when surgery is over."
				O: T 99⁸, P. 88, R. 18, B.P. 124/78. I.V. infusing ® ante cubital space. Operative area has been prepped.
				A: Expected preop apprehension
				P: Will follow routine preop orders and preop teaching plan.
				I: Recovery room explained; coughing, turning, deep breathing & leg exercises explained & demonstrated. Pt. told that pain medication will be available postop and to request at onset of pain. Medicated and prepared for surgery.
	5 PM			E: Understands C.T. & D.B. & exercises — successfully returned demonstration. Med effective — pt. drowsy. Relaxed on departure for O.R.
				M. Reilly, RN
12/16/77	8 PM	1	Appendectomy	S: "My stomach hurts."
				O: Holding abdomen, knees flexed. Voided 200 cc. Incisional dressing dry.
				A: Condition stable — expected postop pain. Vital signs stable (see flowsheet)
				P: Follow pt. care plan.
				I: Routines done. Medicated.
				E: Pain controlled with medication. Sleeping
				M. Reilly, RN
12/17/77	6 AM	1	Appendectomy	S: "uncomfortable"
				O: Incisional dressing dry. VS stable. Taking ice chips
				A: Condition stable
				P: Continue post-op plan
				I: Medicated x 2 this shift for pain
				E: Slept at intervals following pain medication
				J. Kraft R.N.

PROGRESS NOTE FORMAT:
S: Subjective data (symptoms)
O: Objective data (measurable signs)
A: Assessment (conclusion)

P: Plan — immediate or future
I: Intervention — nursing action
E: Evaluation — effectiveness or ineffectiveness of intervention
R: Revision — change care plan appropriately

PATIENT PROGRESS NOTES

DATE	TIME	NO.	PROBLEM	
12/17/77	1 PM	1	APPENDECTOMY	S: SOME DISCOMFORT.
				O: WALKED IN ROOM WITH ASSISTANCE THIS AM.
				A: CONDITION PROGRESSING AS EXPECTED
				P: FOLLOW SAME PLAN.
				G. Nice, R.N.
12/17/77	1 PM	3	DIABETES	S: HUNGRY
			MELLITUS	O: URINE REDUCTIONS HAVE REMAINED NEG.
				FOR SUGAR AND ACETONE. LIQUID ADA
				BREAKFAST AND LUNCH. ORAL HYPOGLYCEMIC
				AGENT GIVEN THIS AM. I.V. TERMINATED.
				BLOOD SUGAR 120
				A: CONDITION CONTROLLED.
				P: WILL CONTINUE PLAN AND REQUEST
				DIABETIC NURSE SPECIALIST TO ASSESS
				PATIENT'S KNOWLEDGE OF D.M. 3RD OR
				4TH POST OP DAY.
				G. Nice, R.N.
12/18/77	10³⁰	1	Appendectomy	S: Minimal discomfort.
				O: No incisional drainage. Has been
				walking in hall.
				A: Post op condition as expected.
				P: Continue with plan.
				I: Instructed in cleansing incision
				and dressing change.
				E: Patient was not afraid to look
				at wound. She will demonstrate
				incisional care tomorrow.
				M. Adams, LPN
12/19/77	2 PM	3	DIABETES	S: No problem with management of diet & medications.
			MELLITUS	O: Diabetic 10 yrs. - verbalized basic definition of
				diabetes; purpose, dosage & side effects of Orinase;
				dietary restrictions & symptoms of hypo &
				hyperglycemia.
				A: Excellent knowledge of disease & management
				P: See no need for additional follow-up.
				P. Swat, R.N.

PROGRESS NOTE FORMAT:
S: Subjective data (symptoms)
O: Objective data (measurable signs)
A: Assessment (conclusion)

P: Plan — immediate or future
I: Intervention — nursing action
E: Evaluation — effectiveness or ineffectiveness of intervention
R: Revision — change care plan appropriately

list, and care plan.

Have you noticed that some POMR entries don't include the IER portion of the SOAPIER format? That's because it isn't always necessary. Sometimes you have nothing to record after those letters, as you can see in the example. But even if that's the case, always include all the letters SOAP in your POMR notes, even if you must leave the S data blank. And be sure to sign your name after each entry, because other health-team professionals will be writing on the same record.

Making flow sheets work for you

Where do flow sheets fit into all this? They provide a way to document repetitive tasks that must be implemented. And that makes them valuable to you, no matter which system of record-keeping you use.

But, flow sheets have other important functions, besides the one I just mentioned. In addition, they:
- keep all routine measurements in one place
- enable you to make a quick comparison of measurements
- provide you with a prompter for care, if you're uncertain about which observations to make
- serve as a legal record to protect you, your patient, or your hospital, if the need arises.

Fortunately for all of us, we can design flow sheets that meet any need; for example, flow sheets designed around a specific disease or problem, so all the necessary procedures and observations can be quickly recorded on it. You can also design a flow sheet suited for the needs of a specific unit in the hospital for instance, Ob/Gyn or ICU.

No matter what kind of flow sheet you use, don't get confused about its purpose. Never get into the habit of redocumenting everything you write on your flow sheet into your narrative or SOAP notes. All you really need to do is summarize your findings, if they're pertinent — or write your impression of them. For example, you might write the following note as a summary: "In the past 8 hours, the patient's blood pressure has ranged from 60/40 to 110/70. It is currently 108/70, and has stabilized."

Sometimes, of course, you needn't write a summary about your flow sheet data. But you can still refer to it on your progress notes. All you have to do is write "See flow sheet," wherever the data seems pertinent.

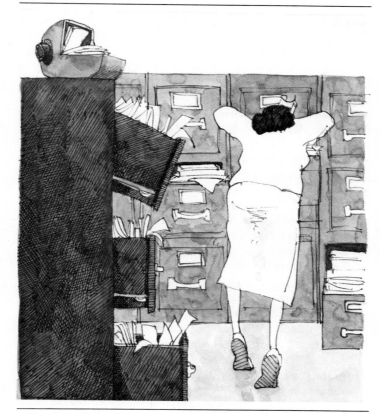

Making the most of flow sheets
If you find yourself foundering in a sea of paper when trying to assess your patient's progress, maybe you're not using his flow sheet effectively. For example, the most efficient way to get a clear picture of how medications are affecting him is to check the flow sheet data.

The graphic arrangement of a flow sheet can help you evaluate the following:
• Relationship between anticoagulant administration and clotting times
• Effectiveness of antibiotic therapy as shown by vital signs changes
• Effect of diuretic therapy on urinary output and weight
• Relationship between insulin administration and fractional urines and blood sugars
• Effects of antineoplastic drug therapy on bone marrow production as shown by blood count results.

Review all the data on your flow sheet before you write your progress notes. If you don't, you may overlook something significant. Remember, part of your responsibility is to read and evaluate all flow sheet findings — and document what you've learned.

Here are some other nursing tips before I close my discussion on flow sheets: Keep them at the patient's bedside. This saves extra steps for you, and may prevent you from forgetting to enter important measurements. Always write your initials after each entry you make.. Then code your initials to your name on the back of the sheet.

Summing up SOAP
Now you know how to write POMR progress notes for your patients. But I realize that some of you don't use the POMR

system in your hospital — which is why I've written Chapter 10. That's where you'll learn how to write better source-oriented progress notes — a valuable skill no matter what system you use.

Keep Mary Anthony's case in mind as you proceed to Chapter 10. But first, review some of the important facts you've learned about writing POMR progress notes:

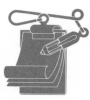

Remember these important rules about writing POMR progress notes:

1. **In POMR progress notes, write separate SOAPIER entries for each problem you've identified on the patient's problem list.**
2. **Each SOAPIER entry must have more than the date and time next to it; it must also have the name and number of the problem it relates to.**
3. **Even if you have no subjective data to relate, write the letter *S* after your entry anyway. Then write why you were unable to get the information.**
4. **You can collect *O* data by using your senses, taking vital signs, or from laboratory tests and X-rays.**
5. **Your *A* data indicates what's going on with your patient. But remember, you can say you don't know what's going on, because *sometimes* you won't be sure.**
6. **In the *P* part of your entry, document what you plan to do about your patient's problem, now or in the future.**
7. **Next to the letter *I* in your entry, document your intervention and be certain it never leaves what you've done up to the reader's imagination.**
8. **In the *E* part of your entry, document your patient's response to your intervention, either positive or negative.**
9. **Use *R* on your notes when the patient's response is not what you expect, and then document how you will revise the plan.**
10. **Use flow sheets to serve these important functions:**
    - **provide a way to document repetitive tasks.**
    - **keep all routine measurements in one place.**
    - **enable you to make a quick comparison of measurements.**
    - **provide you with a prompter for care.**
    - **serve as a legal record to protect you, your patient, or your hospital.**

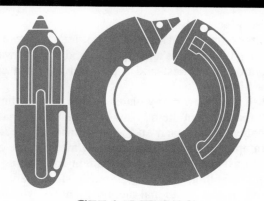

CHARTING
YOUR PATIENT'S PROGRESS
How to use the source-oriented system

BY MARY M. REILLY, RN, BSN

DO YOU USE THE source-oriented system to keep medical records? Then you know the special problems you have keeping track of a patient's progress. Each health-team group documents what they've done in a separate section of the record, and it takes time to link them all together.

For example, you document in the nurses' notes; physical therapists document in their physical therapy notes; and doctors document in their progress notes. If you want to know what's been done for a patient on a specific day, you have to look in three separate sections of the record.

Communication can be difficult

Obviously, this makes communication difficult between you and other health-team professionals — because everyone's busy providing basic care. No one has the time needed to consistently sort through another group's progress notes, so they neglect doing it.

How unfortunate this is, because each professional group needs to know what the other groups are doing. You must know how the patient's responding — not only to *your* care, but to the care of others within the hospital.

Review everyone's notes

Why is this so important? To illustrate, let's suppose you're caring for a patient who's a paraplegic, and you're aware that an occupational therapist and a physical therapist are also caring for him.

How will you know if any plans need to be coordinated, if you don't review all of them? How will you know what to add to your patient's care plan and what to discontinue?

For example, imagine that over a few months, the occupational therapist has brought your patient from being *totally* dependent in eating, to being *partially* dependent. If you haven't read the occupational therapist's notes, you may still be providing total assistance to your patient when he eats. And by doing so, you'd interrupt his progress towards independence.

Or suppose the physical therapist wrote a note on the record, asking you to remind your patient to do certain strengthening exercises. If you didn't read that note, you'd never remind your patient about this important part of his care.

But, isn't communication a two-way process? Yes, those other health-team members must also take time to read your notes. After all, you have plans and requests they should be aware of, too.

All this coordination requires effort on everyone's part, but the rewards are great. The patient receives better care and, of course, he has top priority.

Laying the foundation

Now before I explain exactly how to document your patient's progress using the source-oriented system, let me review the foundation you must build on:
- your initial assessment
- your identification of the patient's problems
- your patient care plan.

As you learned in Chapter 4, you'll need to get a complete assessment of your patient's condition before you can begin to care for him properly. And the guidelines you follow to get this assessment will probably be the same whether you use the source-oriented or problem-oriented system.

What will differ in the source-oriented system is the way you'll document your findings after the assessment. Instead of writing a formal problem list, as you do immediately after assessment in the POMR system, you will determine your nursing diagnoses and put them on the Kardex.

Think back to Chapter 1; it explains how you determine your nursing diagnosis. You make a nursing diagnosis when you identify any problem that interferes with the patient's state of well-being.

Once you've made your nursing diagnosis, you can begin to plan your patient's care (see Chapter 7). To do this properly, you must first review all the data you've collected in your initial assessment.

What to consider
Always consider these three phases of patient care when you write your care plans:
- what observations to make and how often
- what nursing measures to take; when and how to do them
- what to teach or tell the patient and/or his family before he's discharged.

As you already know from Chapter 7, this simple set of guidelines will help you write a better care plan, because it'll force you to be *specific*. But, it'll also help you to *document* the implementation of the plan, because it indicates *exactly* what you should write.

Getting started
Remember how I discussed the case of Mary Anthony to help you understand how to write POMR progress notes (see Chapter 9). Well, now we'll look at her case again, so you can understand how to write source-oriented progress notes. As you know, in the source-oriented system, your notes about Ms. Anthony will be separate from those of the other health-team professions. And you'll write them chronologically — in a narrative style.

Nursing tip: Since some of the tasks or procedures in her care plan are repetitive, you'll probably also record data on a flow sheet. You learned how to use flow sheets, and why they're valuable, in Chapter 9.

Since source-oriented notes are written in narrative style, you won't use the strict SOAP format discussed in Chapter 9. However, you should avoid discussing several problems in a single paragraph, as illustrated in the following example:

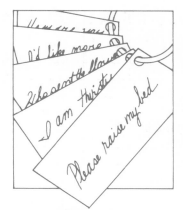

Conversation cards
If you have patients who can't communicate properly, such as those with aphasia or a tracheostomy, here's a way to help them. Write messages, such as "I am thirsty," "Please raise my bed," "I want a drink of water," on index cards. Then punch holes in the cards and attach them to a large key ring so they'll be easy to locate. Patients can quickly communicate their needs and wishes simply by showing you the appropriate card.

You could make several sets of cards for specific times. For example, mealtime cards might include such messages as "I'd like more coffee" and "Please butter my bread." Cards for visiting hours might say "Is there any mail?" "Who sent the flowers?" You can make other cards to meet a particular patient's needs.

NAME _Mary Anthony_

AGE _45_

DATE	TIME	
12/16/77	4 PM	Pt. c/o pain in RLQ – operative area prepped. Nervous about surgery. Sub Q insulin given ; postop teaching done. Temp – 99° – urine sent to lab. Concerned about diabetes.
	5 PM	to O.R. M. Reilly, RN

Instead, discuss each of Ms. Anthony's problems in a separate paragraph, as I've done in her correctly written source-oriented progress notes on page 135.

Organize your thoughts before you write anything. Then your narrative paragraph will be coherent. If you have difficulty deciding what to say in your note, go back to the nursing orders in the patient's care plan. They'll serve as a guideline for documentation, because they list exactly what you're supposed to do for your patient, what you're supposed to observe, and what you're supposed to teach.

If you still have difficulty organizing your thoughts, use the questions listed below as an added guideline. Ask yourself:

• What has my patient said that's significant to the problem I want to discuss in this paragraph?
• What have I seen that relates to this problem?
• What do I really think is happening?
• What do I plan to do about it?
• What have I already done?
• How has my patient responded?

Don't ever forget to ask yourself the last question, because *documenting patient response to care is essential*. It's the only way you can properly evaluate his care plan and determine if it's effective — or if it needs to be replaced with a *better* plan.

When to document

How many times a day do you write on the patient's source-oriented progress notes? Once every hour? Or do you write one paragraph each shift? Or — worse — whenever you think about it?

DATE	TIME	
12/16/77	4 PM	Pt. c/o pain in R L Q and states she's nervous about surgery. Knees are flexed, color pale, and pt. diaphoresing. R.R. procedure explained; pt. took the medication for pain will be available postop, upon request. Taught to turn, cough and deep breathe, while splinting operative site. Leg exercises explained — pt. returned demonstration. Shave prep explained and pt. prepped from nipple line to mid thigh. I. J. of D5W absorbing in ® ante cubital space at 100cc/hr. Pt. concerned about effect of her diabetes on surgery. Reassured that she is a no greater surgical risk. Fractional urines neg/neg. Regular insulin 20 u sub q in Ⓛ arm.
	4:30 PM	Preop — Nembutal 15 mg. I.M. in upper outer quadrant ® buttock. Demerol 50 mg ⟩ I.M. in upper outer quadrant Atropine 0.4 mg ⟩ Ⓛ buttock) Contact lenses in container at bedside.
	5 PM	Pt. drowsy — to O.R. M Reilly, RN

Most hospitals have a specific policy stating when you should record notes. And, as you'd expect, this policy varies from hospital to hospital. *Some say you should write whenever you have something meaningful to record,* which, of course, can be anytime at all.

When your hospital's policy dictates that you document notes on a regular time schedule, you may find yourself writing notes that are repetitious and meaningless. You realize that you're documenting merely to satisfy policy requirements — rather than documenting because you have something important to say.

If you sense this happening, go back and review the following information about your patient: his initial assessment data, his problems, and his care plan. Then relate your documentation more specifically to these three elements of the nursing process. *Never blame policy requirements for poor documentation.*

Unless you're instructed otherwise, write on your patient's progress notes whenever you've observed:

• *a change in his condition* (progression, regression, or addition of new problems). Be specific when you describe the change. Don't say something vague like "condition is improving." Use words that'll help others *visualize* how the patient's improved; for example, "patient is able to ambulate full length of hall."

• *his response to a treatment or a medication.* For example, "medication has not relieved the pain."

• *a lack of change in his condition.* For example, "no change in size or condition of leg ulcer after 5 days of treatment." Remember, to make a note like this meaningful, you must have previously recorded the ulcer's exact measurement and its condition at the start of treatment.

• *his response to specific teaching.* For example, "patient returned demonstration of wound care, and verbalized how often it had to be done (3x daily)."

What to document
Now that I've discussed how and when you should document, let's consider *what* you should document. Always write your notes in specific, descriptive terms. In other words, document exactly what you've heard, observed, inspected, done, or taught. Include any measurements you have made; for exam-

ple, the size of a decubitus ulcer or the size of a palpated lymph node.

Think of your notes as a camera that takes the patient's picture. Be so specific that anyone who reads your notes will be able to see that patient *through your words.*

Avoid using vague terms that can be interpreted in more than one way by the people who'll read your notes. For example, don't record words like these: good, normal, adequate, improving, better, worse, or sufficient.

Suppose you write "adequate output," for example, on the progress notes of a patient with a bladder infection. One person might look at your note and say, "Oh, that must be approximately 1000 ml of urine." Another might say that it means more like 1300 to 1500 ml of urine. Before you write a narrative note, think about the point you want to make by documenting. What do you want to say about your patient? Try to express it so plainly that anyone who reads your note will have a clear understanding of your meaning.

Study the notes I've written to describe Mary Anthony's progress (see page 139). My brief descriptive phrases say as much or more than lengthy sentences.

Always review each of your patient's problems as you consider what to document in the progress notes. For example, if you noticed any change in Ms. Anthony's condition, or she developed new problems, you'd document the change. Suppose, at first, she was afraid to move around after her appendectomy. But when you cared for her today, she was confident and independent. That is certainly a change that should be recorded.

Suppose the nurse on a previous shift documented a change in Ms. Anthony's condition? For example, the appearance of a new symptom. Be sure to comment on that symptom in your progress notes with significant information. If you *don't* comment on the recorded change, *it will look like you never even read the note.* And, of course, the nurse who wrote it won't have any idea how the patient's condition progressed — or deteriorated — when she wasn't on duty.

It may be familiar, but is it significant?

Now let's look at some common phrases we're tempted to use when we document and see if they're worth writing. The first phrase that comes to my mind is "dressings dry and intact."

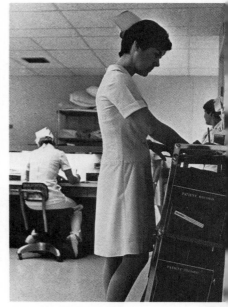

Knowing when to write
Always write on your patient's progress notes when you observe:
• a change in his condition, or the addition of a new problem
• lack of change in condition
• patient's response to treatment or medication
• patient's response to teaching.

For the record
Here's a charting tip that may help you to avoid a possible legal problem: When a note gets written on the wrong chart, draw a line through the note and mark it "Error —wrong chart." *Be sure to sign it, and don't make the line so heavy that the note becomes illegible.*

If you work in an average medical/surgical unit — with patients like Ms. Anthony — you probably see this entered in records day after day. And yet in the majority of patients' records (including Ms. Anthony's), this information isn't significant.

What is significant, however, is what's *under her dressing*: for example, her wound and how it looks. Is it healing? Is it reddened? Is there drainage? Is there an odor? Is there a separation? These are the observations you should document on Ms. Anthony's progress notes (see page 139). The only time you'd find it appropriate to write "dressing dry and intact" is when you've been instructed *not* to remove the initial dressing or inspect the wound.

Another familiar phrase you might be tempted to use in a patient's progress notes is "up and about with no complaints." Now read that carefully. What does it tell you? If your patient has been ambulatory since admission — and everyone knows it — why must it be repeated day after day, shift after shift? As for having "no complaints," have you taken the time to really talk and listen to your patient?

Be careful with words

Never cushion observations or conclusions with words like "seems to be" or "appears to be." For example, don't write "patient seems to be confused," or "patient appears to be congested."

Somewhere along the way, many of us were taught that these words help protect us from documentation errors. In reality, what's happened is that these phrases have made us look uncertain and unsure. So please eliminate them as word choices whenever you document.

Nursing tip: The only time it's appropriate to use the words "appears to be" is in the note "patient appears to be sleeping." Obviously, you can't tell if your patient is really sleeping by just looking at her.

Pretend your words are a camera. Use them to help others "see" your patient.

Some further reminders

Now before you go on to the chapter on how to write a discharge summary, review what you've learned in our discussion.

NURSES NOTES

NAME Mary Anthony

AGE 45

DATE	TIME	
12/16/77	8:00 PM	Returned from R.R.- dressing dry - BP 124/80 T. 99.8
		I.V. of D₅W absorbing well at 25 gtts/minute
		c/o pain at incision site. Knees flexed M. Reilly, RN
	8:30 PM	Demerol 75 mg IM B Frick R.N.
	9:30 PM	Pain controlled with medication -
		Encouraged to turn and cough
	11 PM	BP 124/78 Dressing dry. Sleeping.
		M. Reilly, RN
12/17/77	12 AM	Sleeping at intervals. c/o incisional pain. Dressing dry
		T 99.6 BP 124/78
	12:30 AM	Demerol 75 mg IM J. Kraft R.N
	4:00 AM	IV absorbing well. Voided 400 ml pale yellow urine
		VS stable (see flowsheet) Sleeping at intervals. Pt
		turned and coughed while splinting incision
	6:15 AM	c/o incisional pain. Demerol 75 mg IM J. Kraft R.N.
12/17/77	8:30 AM	LIQUID ADA DIET TAKEN WELL – URINE REDUCTION Neg. FOR S AND A.
		DRESSING DRY – NO BLEEDING NOTED – VS STABLE. PT. COMPLAINED
		OF INCISIONAL DISCOMFORT. IV DISCONTINUED.
	10:30 AM	MEDICATED FOR PAIN – THEN PT. AMBULATED IN ROOM c̄ ASSISTANCE.
	12:00 NOON	LIQUID ADA LUNCH TOLERATED WELL. LEG EXERCISES COMPLETED.
		DRESSING CHANGE BY DOCTOR. NO DRAINAGE FROM INCISION.
	3:00 PM	SLEPT AT INTERVALS. WILL CONTACT DIABETIC NURSE SPECIALIST
		TO EVALUATE PATIENT'S KNOWLEDGE OF D.M. G. Rice, R.N.
12/17/77	4:00 PM	Demerol 75 mg. IM. M. Adams, LPN.
	5:00 PM	OOB Ambulating in room – Voiding QS
		VS stable – Progressing as expected.
	9:00 PM	Incisional discomfort -
	9:15 PM	Demerol 75 mg. IM
	11:00 PM	Sleeping M. Adams, LPN
12/18/77	3:00 AM	Pt slept well till now. c/o incisional discomfort.
		Dressing checked. Incision healing well; no drainage
		BP 120/80. Repositioned. Back care
	3:30	Demerol 50 mg IM given. Sleeping J. Kraft R.N.
12/18/77	10:30 AM	Minimal discomfort. Has been walking in hall. Soft
		ADA diet tolerated well.
	12:00 N.	Instructed in cleaning incision and dressing change.
		Will return demonstration 12/19/78 M. Adams, LPN.

Remember these rules about documenting source-oriented progress notes:

1. Always read the notes written by the other health-team professionals before you write your own.
2. Always be specific.
3. Always be descriptive.
4. Always ask yourself these questions before you document:
   What have you heard?
   What have you seen?
   What do you think?
   What will you do?
   What have you done?
   How did the patient respond?
5. Always write on your patient's progress notes when you observe:
   • a change in his condition, or the addition of a new problem
   • lack of change in condition
   • patient's response to treatment or medication
   • patient's response to teaching.
6. Always use the flow sheet to document repetitious procedures or measurements and summarize that information in the narrative note.
7. Always write separate narrative paragraphs about each problem that you may be documenting about at one time.
8. Always avoid vague words like "normal," "good," or "adequate."
9. Always read the notes recorded by nurses on other shifts and make further comments on their findings to maintain continuity of care.
10. Always sign your name after each entry.

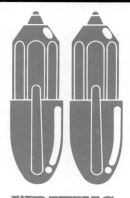

WRITING
THE DISCHARGE SUMMARY
What to tell your patient

BY MARY M. REILLY, RN, BSN

DO YOU KNOW HOW TO WRITE a proper discharge summary? You should, because it's one part of the patient's record that's taken on new importance for you in recent years — and rightly so.

Not long ago, you wrote everything you wanted to say about a departing patient at the end of his record in a brief note. And that's precisely what it was — a note — and nothing more.

Consider this discharge note, an example of what I mean:

Date	Time	Progress notes
5/23/78	10³⁰ AM	*Pt discharged via wheelchair to family* *J. Jones R.N.*

It doesn't say much, does it? For instance, it hasn't told you what condition the patient's in, what medications he took home with him, when he was scheduled to see the doctor again, or what he was taught.

Today a discharge note like this is no longer adequate. Instead, you write a complete summary of your patient's hospitalization — describing what occurred to him during that time and what you did about it.

What's in; what's out
Does that mean you write a day-to-day account of everything that happened? No — just the *significant highlights* from your patient's hospitalization. In other words, describe what your patient was like on admission and what he's like now at discharge. When necessary, include notes that refer the reader back to the progress notes or flow sheets, but don't recopy everything that's happened for the summary.

Always review your patient's care plan before you write your discharge summary — to make sure you discuss everything listed on it. Then check over the flow sheets, so you can document the range of significant measurements.

For example, you'd decide which measurements *related* to the problems discussed in your summary — then you'd write something similar to the following:

Date	Time	Progress notes
		On admission, pt's B.P. was 150/106. At discharge it is 130/92. The highest reading during this hospitalization was 160/100 (See flow sheet)

Never repeat day-to-day flow-sheet measurements in the summary. But, if one day's measurement is particularly significant, copy that and write a note saying exactly where to find it on the flow sheet.

Suppose your patient is being transferred to another hospital, nursing home, or rehabilitation center. Try to think of the data that will be most helpful to the health-care professionals in these settings and include it. Make sure they get a copy of the discharge summary when your patient is transferred. This will assure continuity of care for him, which always affects the quality.

Plan ahead
Obviously, you won't *write* your patient's discharge summary ahead of time. But writing is only *part* of your responsibility to the patient. *You begin making plans for his discharge the day he's admitted.*

For example, you'll get some idea of what you have to teach him before discharge when you make your initial assessment

— provided, of course, you did it properly. Ask yourself:
- What should I teach this patient about his illness or condition?
- What should I tell him about his medication?
- What should I teach him about his dietary restrictions, if any?
- What must he learn about the procedures he's expected to perform at home?
- If his activities are to be restricted, how can I help him fit these restrictions into his life-style?

Make each encounter meaningful

As soon as you've determined your patient's educational needs, make plans to fulfill them. But don't wait till the last minute to teach him what he needs to know, make it a gradual, ongoing process. Then by the time he's discharged, you'll have some idea how much he understands. And, of course, you'll document this on his discharge summary — so everyone will know which points he's still confused about, and which he understands.

Where do you write your summary?

Now, let's discuss where you write your patient's discharge summary. Do you write it on a printed form, or at the end of your patient's progress notes?

The summary always appears at the end of the patient's progress notes. And in most cases, you write it out yourself. What varies is the *style* it's written in, and this depends on the type of record-keeping you use.

For example, if you have the POMR system in your hospital, you'll write your discharge summary in the style of a SOAP or SOAPIER note. Then it will be consistent with the rest of your progress notes, and easily understandable.

However, if you use the source-oriented system, you'll write your summary in narrative paragraphs. Or — as an alternative — you can put the same information on a printed discharge form and use *that* to conclude your patient's record.

A word of warning, though: Make sure the printed form you use has a place for *all* the information you need to document about the patient at discharge. If it doesn't, you will still have to write a *separate summary* to include everything at the end of your progress notes.

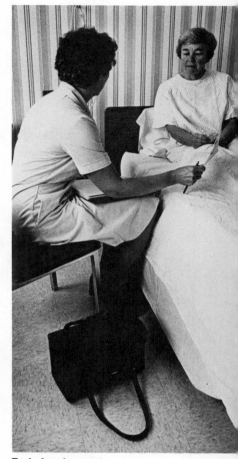

Early involvement
If you anticipate that your patient will need the services of a visiting nurse after discharge, contact her as soon as possible. She should interview the patient before her discharge.

How to write a POMR discharge summary

I've told you how discharge summaries vary in style; now let me explain exactly how to write one if your hospital uses the problem-oriented system of record-keeping.

As you already know, you'll make all your entries in the SOAP or SOAPIER style — which was explained in Chapter 9. Each of the patient's problems will be numbered and have its own SOAP summary, provided that problem is still active.

But what do you do if one or more of these problems has been resolved by that time? You still list the problem — and number it — in the discharge summary. However, you write that it was resolved and list the date it was resolved, so the reader can refer to the progress notes.

For example, here's a discharge summary entry written about a patient who had a postop bladder infection for a few days:

Date	Time	No.	Problem	Progress notes
5/3/78	10 AM	5	Bladder infection	Resolved 4/29/78 (see progress notes) J. Kraft RN

To get a clear picture of how a POMR discharge summary should look, see page 145. It was written for Mary Anthony, who was discussed at length in Chapters 9 and 10. If you need to review her case, see her assessment sheet, problem list, and initial plan in the appendix. Then refer to her POMR progress notes in Chapter 9.

Writing the patient instruction sheet

What about a written sheet of instructions for Mary to take home? You can't give her a copy of her complete POMR discharge summary. So you'll have to prepare something for her alone, which will tell her all she needs to know about her condition, medication, diet, and activity restrictions.

You can do this in two ways:

• Use a patient instruction sheet, such as the one illustrated on page 149. Then pull out all the information your patient needs to know from your discharge summary and write it on the sheet, in a way that he'll understand.

PATIENT PROGRESS NOTES

NAME _Mary Anthony_

AGE _45_

DATE	TIME	NO.	PROBLEM	
12/20/77		1	Appendectomy (discharge summary)	S: Admitted 12/16/77 with severe RLQ pain. Following surgery, postop pain for several days. Now feels good—ready to go home.
				O: Incision is clean and dry. Pt. ambulatory with assistance for 48 hours and has not received a narcotic in that time. Discomfort controlled with Darvon. BP pre- and postop remained 116/70 and 126/84 (see flow sheet).
				A: Wound healing. Condition stable throughout postop period.
				P: Pt. will be discharged to family.
				I: Instructed pt. to cleanse wound daily with Betadine; no dressing. Avoid heavy household tasks (i.e. scrubbing floors). Light tasks are permitted (i.e. dishes). Obstain from sexual activity for 3 weeks. Call for appointment with surgeon in 2-3 weeks. Has prescription for Darvon 65 mg for discomfort. Instruction sheet given.
				E: Pt. successfully demonstrated incision care and verbalized instructions.
				M. Reilly, RN
12/20/77		3	diabetes mellitus (discharge summary)	S: Comfortable with our management of disease
				O: NPO on admission with D5W I.V. at 100 cc/hr. Progressed postop from ADA liquid to general ADA 1800 cal diet. All urine reductions were neg for S & A. Given insulin (Sub-Q) prior to and for first postop day. Then resumed Orinase 0.25 g. b.i.d. Knowledge assessment completed by clinical specialist; see note 12/19/77.
				A: Disease process controlled with medication and diet.
				P: Discharge on medication and diet. Pt. will schedule appointment with family doctor in 2 months.
				M. Reilly, RN

PROGRESS NOTE FORMAT:
S: Subjective data (symptoms)
O: Objective data (measurable signs)
A: Assessment (conclusion)

P: Plan — immediate or future
I: Intervention — nursing action
E: Evaluation — effectiveness or ineffectiveness of intervention
R: Revision — change care plan appropriately

NURSES NOTES

NAME _Mary Anthony_

AGE _45_

DATE	TIME	
12/20/77	discharge summary	Appendicitis
		Pt. admitted 12/16/77 with severe R L Q pain – To surgery 12/16/77 for appendectomy. Pt. tolerated procedure well. Postop vital signs stable (see flow sheet). She has been ambulatory for 48 hours and has not required a narcotic in that time. Incisional discomfort controlled with Darvon 65 mg (prescription sent home with pt.) Incision clean and dry. Pt. instructed to clean wound daily with Betadine. No dressing. Pt. returned demonstration of wound care. Pt. to avoid heavy household tasks (i.e. running sweeper, scrubbing floors) Light tasks permitted (dusting, dishes) Abstain from sexual activity for 3 weeks. Call for an appt. with surgeon 2-3 weeks. Pt. verbalized instruction. Instruction sheet given.
		Diabetes mellitus
	discharge summary	Pt. comfortable with management of disease. Postop progressed from ADA liquid diet to 1800 cal ADA. Urine reductions have been neg/neg – while NPO and I.V. running. Pt. was given reg insulin subcutaneously on 2/17/77 Orinase .25 g b.i.d. resumed. Evaluation of knowledge done by diabetic nurse specialist. See note 12/19/77 Pt. to schedule appt. with internist in 2 months.
		M. Reilly, RN

• List all the patient's active problems on a sheet and number them. Then pull out all the information your patient needs to know about each of his problems and write it after the problem names. Write in clear, easy-to-understand terms. Do not use the letters SOAP.

Remember this: No matter how you prepare an instruction sheet for your patient, document that you've done so next to the I on your SOAPIER discharge summary.

How to write a source-oriented discharge summary

Now, let's talk about source-oriented discharge summaries. As I said before, if you use this record-keeping system, you'll write your patient's summary in narrative paragraphs at the end of his progress notes.

Follow the same procedure you used writing his progress notes. Avoid discussing several problems in a single paragraph. Instead, summarize each problem in a *separate paragraph or paragraphs*. To organize your thoughts about each problem, before you write your summary, ask yourself these questions:

• What are the patient's symptoms at this time — or how does she say she feels? (Subjective data)

• What are the patient's signs at this time or what factual data have you gathered by observing and inspecting her? (Objective data)

• What conclusion have you come to about the patient's problem at this time? (Assessment)

• What do you plan to do about his problem now, or after he leaves the hospital? (Plan of care)

• What have you already done for your patient, relative to this problem? (Intervention)

• What was the outcome of your intervention? Was it effective or ineffective? (Evaluation)

• How will you change the patient's care plan, if your intervention hasn't proved successful? (Revision)

Same categories, different systems

As you can see, you use the same categories to organize your notes as you do in the POMR system. The only difference is style. When you write a source-oriented discharge summary, you don't list the letters SOAPIER before each entry. You simply write the information next to the problem name.

For an example of a source-oriented discharge summary, written in this way, see Mary Anthony's summary on page 146.

What kind of patient instruction sheet?
Obviously, you can't give your patient a copy of her complete source-oriented discharge summary — any more than you could give her a copy of her POMR summary. So you'll prepare a separate patient instruction sheet, like the one on the opposite page, listing everything she should know.

Consider your patient's educational level when you write it, and use words she can understand. Then document that you've given her an instruction sheet at the end of your progress notes' summary.

Talking things over
Now, let's discuss what you must teach your patient before his discharge — and how soon you start doing it. Obviously, you don't wait till the morning he's going to leave to tell him all he needs to know. That would be poor planning.

Instead, you start planning his discharge on admission and teach him a little at a time. Then you have more opportunities to assess his understanding level, and reinforce what he doesn't comprehend immediately.

On page 147, I mentioned the questions you should ask yourself when you're determining a patient's educational needs. And these questions relate the specific categories, usually included on every patient instruction sheet (see opposite page).

For example, before he goes home, the average patient will need instruction from you about:
- the medications he'll be taking
- the procedures he's expected to perform
- his dietary restrictions, if any
- his activity restrictions, if any
- his follow-up care.

What to tell your patient about his medications
First, consider the medications your patient will be taking after discharge. You'll list these on his instruction sheet, along with dosage and the prescribed time schedule.

But, you must do more than that to teach your patient properly. You must help him work that time schedule into his

PATIENT DISCHARGE INSTRUCTION SHEET

I. DIET:

Your diet will be _1800 cal ADA_

Restrictions: _none. May continue to use diabetic sweets_

II. MEDICATIONS:

Medication	Time to be taken	Possible side effects
Orinase .25 g	Twice a day	rash, headache, ringing in ears indigestion, vomiting, light headedness
Darvon 65mg	One capsule every 3-4 hrs as needed for pain	rash, abdominal cramps, agitation, yellowish skin

Medication which should not be taken: _cough preparations, unless sugarless. Tell your doctor if you are taking any sedatives, tranquilizers, antidepressants, or pain relievers including aspirin_

III. ACTIVITIES:

Your activities:

__X__ may shower

__—__ tub bath

__—__ sponge bath

__X__ climb stairs (limit to twice a day)

__X__ drive a car in 3 weeks

__X__ resume sexual activities in 3 weeks

__X__ other light housework only (dishes + dusting)

IV. FOLLOW-UP CARE:

You should see your physician ___—___ on _Call for an appt. in 2-3 weeks_

V. WOUND CARE:

Your wound should be cared for in the following manner: _Wash incision daily with Betadine_
No dressing. Contact doctor if there is an increase in any drainage (blood or pus) from incision; redness or swelling of incision; or fever

VI. SPECIAL INSTRUCTIONS:

Contact physician if you experience:

1) Unusual pain in legs, back, chest, stomach not controlled by Darvon

2) Fever

3) Chest congestion

4) Persistent vomiting

life-style, so he doesn't have trouble taking his medication as ordered.

For example, let's suppose your patient is scheduled to take his medication 4 times a day. And, throughout his hospital stay, he's received it at 9 a.m., 12 noon, 3 p.m., and 6 p.m. He may think there's something so "special" about those hours that he can't take his medication at any other times. This misconception could make him *skip a dose* when it interfered with his life-style, or — even worse — *double his dosage* to make up for times lost.

To prevent this kind of misunderstanding, explain time schedules to your patient carefully. Read over the section labeled "typical day profile" in his initial assessment sheet. If you see that he'll have trouble taking his medication on schedule, talk it over with him. Help him work out a schedule that he can live with — and that will also be acceptable by the doctor prescribing the medication.

Alert him to the side effects he may experience from his medication, and tell him to call his doctor if he notices any of the symptoms. Giving him a patient teaching card about his medication is a good way to help him remember all he needs to know. I've illustrated the card you'd give Mary Anthony below. But you can see many other examples — and copy them for your own use — in the Nursing Skillbook, GIVING CARDIOVASCULAR DRUGS SAFELY.

DARVON
PATIENT TEACHING AID

Dear Patient:
Here's what you should know about the drug your doctor has prescribed for you. Darvon (propoxyphene) is a nonnarcotic analgesic which will relieve your pain.

Follow these instructions carefully:

1. Take the medication, as prescribed, at the onset of pain. You should feel the full benefit of it in 1 to 2 hours.
2. Tell your doctor first if you also take sedatives, sleep-inducing drugs, tranquilizers, antidepressants, or narcotics.
3. Use caution if you must operate machinery, drive a vehicle, or pilot a plane, since Darvon can impair your mental alertness, coordination, and judgment.
4. Don't drink alcohol when you take Darvon.

Call your doctor immediately if you notice any of the following: extreme drowsiness, lightheadedness, rash, vomiting, abdominal cramps, insomnia, agitation, or jaundice (yellowish skin or sclera).

What to tell your patient about procedures

Now, let's talk about the procedures your patient will be expected to perform when he goes home. In some cases, these may be quite complicated and will require a lot of teaching on your part — from the time of admission.

For example, if you have a patient with colostomy, you may have to teach him to irrigate it. And you'll have to teach him how to care for his stoma, so it doesn't become irritated.

Try to assess your patient's level of understanding before you explain procedures, and tailor your teaching to that level. If you sense that your patient will have trouble grasping your instructions in the time you've allotted, readjust your time schedule and teach more slowly. *Always give your instructions in words the patient can understand.*

Clear up any misconceptions he may have about time schedules. For example, suppose the doctor wants him to apply warm compresses to an ulcerated area 3 times a day. If your patient's life-style is such that he's not home at the same times you applied the compresses in the hospital, he may just forget about them.

Try to foresee these problems in advance, by reading his typical day profile. Then help him fit the necessary procedures into his life-style.

Always consider the possibility that he misunderstands other things about the procedures. For example, suppose you've just explained to him the schedule for warm compresses over the ulcerated area. Go one step further, and discuss the "equipment" he needs to complete the procedure. He may think he needs the 4x4 sterile pads you're using in the hospital, when a clean washcloth will serve as well. Or he may think he needs a special bowl, when any clean bowl in his house will be adequate.

I've known cases where a patient just gave up trying to perform a prescribed procedure because he thought he lacked the necessary equipment. That's why you should consider your patient's setting after he leaves the hospital, and explain how he can adapt the procedure to it.

What to tell your patient about his dietary restrictions

Will your patient have a special diet to follow when he leaves the hospital? If so, go over it in detail with him, or ask the dietician to. Make sure he understands exactly what the diet requires and restricts, and *why he's on it*.

Be very specific when you discuss the restrictions in the diet. For example, if your patient's on a no-salt diet, explain that this restriction involves more than just the table salt he uses — it also restricts the salt he uses for cooking.

Check into his life-style before you discuss his diet with him. Will someone else be planning and cooking his meals? Be sure to include that person in your teaching sessions, so she understands the importance of compliance.

Offer all the help you can by suggesting menus, recipes, and shopping tips. For a good example of a teaching aid you can copy and hand out to patients on fat-controlled diets, see the one in the appendices of the Nursing Skillbook, GIVING CARDIOVASCULAR DRUGS SAFELY.

If you sense the patient will have difficulty staying on his diet for some reason, always get help from the hospital's dietician or the social service department. For example, suppose you realize that your patient won't be able to shop for food or cook his own meals for a while. Ask the social service department to arrange for a homemaker or Meals-On-Wheels.

What to tell your patient about activity restrictions
If your patient has had surgery, he probably must avoid certain activities for a while. For example, he may not be permitted to do any heavy lifting — and maybe he won't even be able to drive his car.

Before you discuss these restrictions with him, find out what his normal activities are. Then be very specific which ones he must avoid, so he has no trouble understanding how the restrictions affect his life-style.

For example, if he can't do any heavy lifting, *relate that restriction to his normal activity pattern*. Don't say that heavy lifting refers to activities like carrying wet laundry if your patient never does housework. By ignoring his normal activity pattern, you may be overlooking some kind of heavy lifting he *does* do. For example, he may be a librarian and lift heavy books all day, as part of his job.

In some cases, your patient's activities will be so restricted that he won't be able to care for himself when he returns home. If so, call the social service department and arrange for help early. Otherwise, your patient's discharge may be delayed while these matters are cared for.

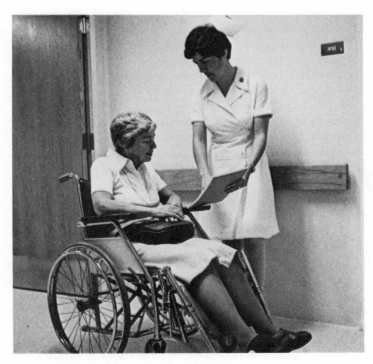

What to tell your patient about follow-up care

Your patient will probably have to return to his doctor for one or more checkups after he leaves the hospital. Make sure he understands why this is important and knows when he's expected to make the appointment.

If he already has a scheduled appointment, write it on his patient instruction sheet. Then talk it over with him to make sure he can keep it. Can he drive himself to the doctor's office or clinic? Or does he need transportation? *Never overlook the possibility that he has no way to get to the doctor's office.* Always check this out and get help for him if it's needed.

Be sure to give your patient a phone number he can call if he has any problems *before* he returns for his checkup. But remind him that his checkup isn't just to take care of problems; he must return even if he's feeling good.

Summarizing the important points

When you've completed teaching your patient all he needs to know before he leaves the hospital, summarize it for him. In a sense, that's his own discharge summary, just like the one you wrote for yourself on his records.

By now, you know that writing a discharge summary involves more than just documenting. No matter what record-keeping system you use, proper discharge planning is the essential first step towards writing a correct summary.

So you won't forget what you've learned in this chapter, I've repeated ten of the most important points below. Review them now before you go on to the next chapter.

Remember these important rules about writing a discharge summary:

1. **Start planning for the patient's discharge from the day of his admission.**
2. **Before you write anything, review his care plan, so that you'll be thorough in your summary.**
3. **Always review the patient's initial assessment form before you plan his discharge, so you can determine what help and education he'll need.**
4. **Review all flow sheets, so you can summarize all significant data onto the discharge summary.**
5. **Don't repeat all the data listed on the flow sheets or progress notes. Just pick out the significant highlights, or the range of pertinent measurements.**
6. **Write a separate SOAP summary or narrative summary for each problem you have dealt with during the patient's hospitalization.**
7. **Always write your SOAP summary or narrative discharge summary at the end of your progress notes.**
8. **Don't use a printed form in place of your narrative discharge summary unless you are sure it provides for all necessary information.**
9. **After you've written a summary for the end of the progress notes, pull out the information the patient needs to know and write it on a separate patient instruction sheet.**
10. **After you give the patient his instruction sheet, document that you've done so in your discharge summary.**

SKILLCHECK 4

1. Which of the following entries should you include after the "O" on your SOAPIER notes?
a) Patient complaining of spasmodic pain in LLQ, occurring ½ hour p.c.
b) Patient experiencing an insulin reaction.
c) Demonstrate colostomy irrigation to patient.
d) Abdomen distended, bowel sounds absent.

2. Your patient draws up an incorrect dosage of insulin into the syringe after you've demonstrated the procedure. Where do you document this information on your problem-oriented medical records?
a) On a flow sheet
b) Next to E on your SOAPIER notes
c) On the problem list
d) Next to P on your SOAPIER notes.

3. Which of the following entries should you include as A data on your POMR progress notes?
a) Patient feels weak and is diaphoretic
b) Uncertain as to cause of rash
c) Make referral to social service department
d) Include wife in dietary teaching program.

4. Which of the following excerpts is an example of proper source-oriented documentation?
a) Patient appears to be confused
b) Vital signs normal following arteriogram
c) Abdominal girth measures 47 inches
d) Wound draining more profusely today.

5. Under what circumstance must you always write an entry on your source-oriented progress notes?
a) When you want to document frequent or repetitious tasks

b) When your patient's condition has changed
c) When A.M. care is completed
d) When you have to add to the problem list.

6. How should you document patient problems on your source-oriented progress notes?
a) Use narrative style and discuss one problem per paragraph.
b) Use a SOAPIER format.
c) Use a narrative care plan format.
d) Use a time sequence to arrange paragraphs which might include several problems.

7. What kind of written instructions should you give your patient before she's discharged?
a) A copy of her complete POMR discharge summary
b) Information your patient needs to know which you've pulled from the discharge summary
c) Patient teaching cards for medications only
d) None, because you will be liable for errors.

8. Philip Jenkins, 43, is to be discharged from your unit. How should you write a POMR discharge summary for him?
a) Write one narrative note summarizing Mr. Jenkin's problems.
b) Fill in a patient instruction sheet and include this on the chart.
c) Write SOAPIER notes summarizing each of Mr. Jenkin's problems at the end of the progress notes. Then give him the information he needs to know on a patient instruction sheet.
d) Briefly describe Mr. Jenkins' general appearance on the progress notes. Also indicate his mode of leaving and disposition of valuables.

(Answers on page 181)

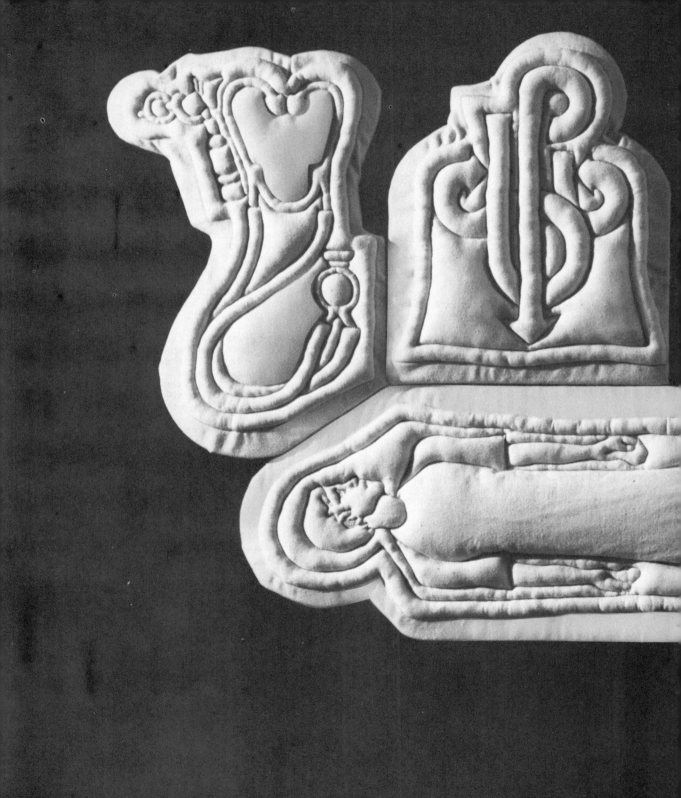

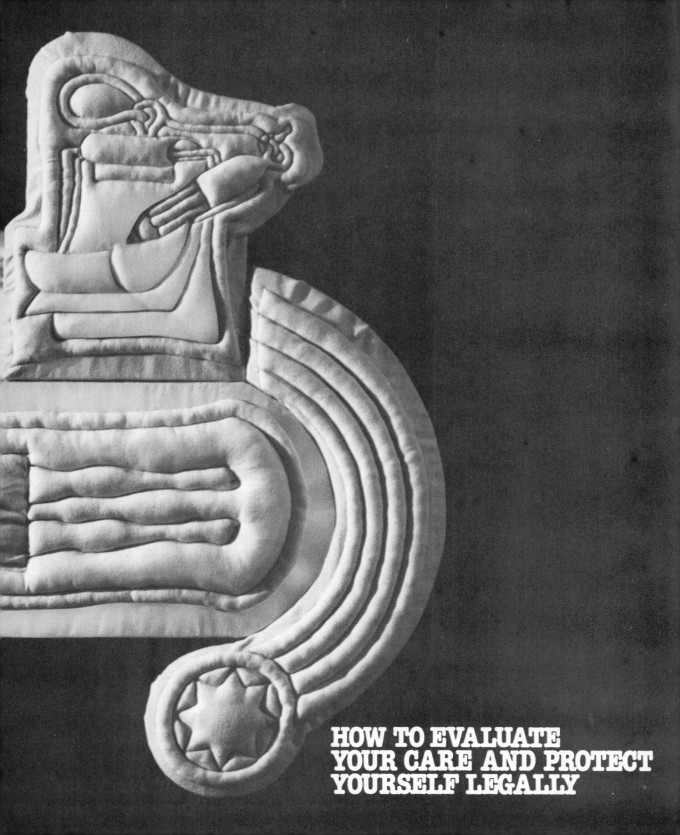

HOW TO EVALUATE
YOUR CARE AND PROTECT
YOURSELF LEGALLY

"Your documentation is
the only proof you have
that your patient was
cared for properly."

"Never let long periods of time
go by without any charting.
It may look like your patient
was neglected during that time."

"A properly written
patient record is your best defense
against legal action."

"Make sure you have
a written policy for everything you do
that may be considered
controversial."

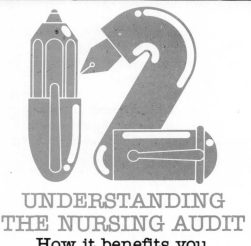

UNDERSTANDING THE NURSING AUDIT
How it benefits you

BY ELLEN K. VASEY, RN, MPH

HOW DO YOU REACT when you hear the words "nursing audit"? Do you feel like you're under a magnifying glass? Do you start worrying about the documentation you've been doing — for fear it'll prove deficient?

Well if these are your reactions, you have the wrong idea about a nursing audit. This systematic evaluation procedure is something you should welcome, because it benefits you, the patient, other health-team professionals, and the hospital.

How it helps
Let's take a look at how it helps. A properly done nursing audit does the following:

• It improves patient care, not only by helping you pinpoint where you fail to carry out the nursing process properly, but by providing you with methods to correct those failures.

• It demonstrates deficiencies in hospital policies and procedures. For example, when expected goals for patient care can't be met because of written or unwritten policies, the audit identifies these policies and gives direction for change.

• It encourages total coordination of health-team planning for patient care.

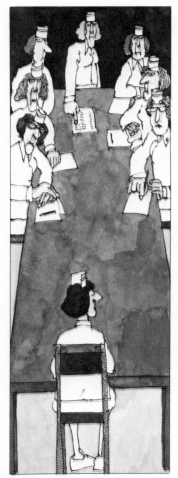

Peer review — not peer pressure
When the audit committee representative pulls charts for an audit committee meeting, do you feel threatened? Do you feel your job's in jeopardy?

Don't! The goal of the audit committee is to help you use your time to your patients' fullest advantage.

• It improves communication between all departments and services by involving everyone in a quality assurance program.

• It provides better documentation of patient care, because it explains exactly what's expected.

• By identifying the strengths and weaknesses of the staff, it provides direction for inservice educational programs that'll help them upgrade the quality of patient care.

• It points out where additional facilities, equipment, or staff are needed.

• By developing criteria and measuring it against actual practice, it provides a way to study particular aspects of patient care.

• It shows both the public and the governing body of the hospital that patient care is being monitored systematically. And it provides a way to evaluate the quality of that care and report on it.

You and the Joint Commission
As you know, the Joint Commission has developed a patient-care audit procedure that enables you to objectively evaluate the patient care you provide — and then determine what *corrective* action is needed if that care is deficient.

To successfully carry out this recommended procedure, your audit committee must do these five things:

• develop the criteria or standards of care that will serve as a measuring stick for the audit of the record. These criteria must not only relate to the topic, but also be well-defined in measurable terms.

• measure retrievable data from patient charts to show when, and how many times, these standards of care are met. By calculating what percentage of patient records meets these standards, the audit committee can determine the quality of care. *Of course, this is true only if the retrievable data reflects an accurate picture of patient care.*

• evaluate records that don't meet the criteria to see why these standards for care are not met. If the failure to meet the criteria is not justified, the audit committee determines the cause and makes plans to correct it.

• develop and act on a plan that will solve the problems interfering with quality care.

• reaudit the records, or do a follow-up study to see if the

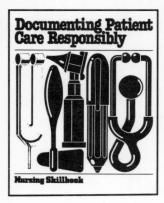

plan was effective. If it wasn't, a new plan must be chosen and implemented.

Three types of criteria

Now let's take a closer look at the audit committee's first step: developing criteria or standards of care.

To do an audit, the committee may develop one or all of these sets of criteria:

• outcome criteria, which focus on the patient and the end result of his care. In setting outcome criteria, the committee first defines the goals the patient should achieve at discharge for his particular illness or surgery. These goals or outcomes must be in measurable terms. Then the committee establishes where on the patient's record you should document the specific information relating to those goals.

• process criteria, which focus on you and the kind of care you give your patients. The audit committee usually scrutinizes your nursing care when a large percentage of outcome criteria is not met or when too many complications occur. When they set process criteria, they outline exactly what you're expected to do to help your patient meet his expected goal.

• structure criteria, which focus on the department and the way it functions. For example, if an outcome audit showed a high percentage of patients sustaining injuries from falls, the committee might decide to look at the safety measures used in that department to see what's causing the problem.

The audit worksheets

As soon as the nursing audit committee has established the basic criteria for the topics they want to study, they put it on worksheets, such as the ones shown on pages 162 and 163.

These worksheets then serve as guidelines for the committee to use throughout the audit procedure. In many hospitals, they are also available for the nursing staff to examine, so you can see exactly what criteria are expected.

Examining the outcome criteria worksheet

To understand how these audit worksheets are set up, turn to page 162 and examine the outcome criteria worksheet prepared for patients like Mary Anthony, who underwent appendectomy.

The audit committee solves a problem
Here's an example of how one audit committee recognized and solved a problem: An investigation showed catheter care was not consistently documented on each shift. Further inquiry revealed catheter care wasn't done because there was no equipment on the unit. Why? No one had time to go to central supply to get it.

The audit committee recommended that day shift obtain three catheter-care kits for each patient with a catheter and place them at the bedside. Problem solved.

OUTCOME AUDIT CRITERIA

Audit Topic: Appendectomy   **Committee:** Nursing Audit   **Date:** October 1978

NO.	ELEMENTS	EXPECTED ALL	NONE	EXCEPTIONS	EXPLANATIONS FOR MEDICAL DATA ANALYST
	Health				
1.	Afebrile	X		None	Normal temp. 100° F. or ↓ (oral) for 24 h prior to discharge. Documented on clinical record.
2.	Pain-free or controlled by oral medication	X		None	No I.M. pain. Med given for 24 h prior to discharge. Documented on med sheet.
3.	Healing incision	X		None	Documented in patient progress notes (O, A) that incision is clean and dry — healing.
	Activity				
4.	Ambulatory	X		Other debilitating disease	Ambulatory without assistance for 24 h prior to discharge. Documented on flow sheet √ data base — activity.
	Knowledge				
5.	Pt. and S.O. received instructions on: Care of incision	X		None	Documented in patient progress notes (1) that patient and S.O. were told and returned demonstration of incisional care.
6.	Activity level	X		None	Doc. by RN on patient progress notes or discharge summary (1) re: activity and/or limitations including stairs, work, driving, and sexual activity.
7.	Return visit	X		None	Doc. by RN in patient progress notes or discharge summary (1) when, where, and who patient is referred for follow-up care.
	Complications				
8.	Wound infection		X	1) Observations of incision 2) Sterile dressings 3) Drainage sent for C/S 4) Notify MD at onset of symptoms also surveillance RN	Temp. ↑ 101° F. 3-5 days postop with reddened, purulent, draining incision with odor. Doc. on graphic/progress notes (O).
9.	Pneumonia (chest congestion)		X	1) Preop instructions 2) Cough, turn, deep-breathe q2h until ambulatory 3) Notify MD and head nurse T.L. or supervisor at onset of symptoms	Cough with congestion, chest rales occurring with temp. ↑ 101° F. Document temperature on graphic/progress notes (O).
10.	Phlebitis at I.V. site			—Discontinue I.V. —Notify I.V. team —Warm compresses to site —Notify MD if extensive	Redness, tenderness, swelling or inflammation at I.V. site — doc. on progress notes.
11.	Other				Return all death charts and any other complications on face sheet.

PROCESS AUDIT CRITERIA

Audit Topic: Lower abdominal surgery   **Committee:** Nursing Audit   **Date:** October 1978

NO.	ELEMENTS	EXPECTED ALL	EXPECTED NONE	EXCEPTIONS	EXPLANATIONS FOR MEDICAL DATA ANALYST
	Assessment Interview				
1.	Pain — site, type	X		None	All documentation in progress notes, flow sheet, vital signs sheet.
2.	Presence or absence of nausea	X		None	
	Observe–Inspect				
3.	Vital signs — temp, pulse, resp, and BP pressure	X		None	
4.	Mental status	X		None	
5.	Skin color	X		None	
6.	Abdominal dressing for presence or absence of drainage	X		No dressing	
	Management				
7.	Turn, cough, deep-breathe q2h til ambulatory	X		None	
8.	Leg exercises q2h til ambulatory				
9.	Dressing q2h for 1st 12 h for hemorrhage	X		No dressing	
10.	Offer pain med q4h	X			

Keeping ahead of the audit
Do you have trouble remembering
to document the nursing care
items that might be audited by
your hospital's quality assurance
committee?

If so, you might want to borrow
an idea currently used at an
eastern hospital: prepare a list of
criteria for various disease
conditions. For each disease,
certain items must be
documented before the patient is
discharged. For example, criteria
for a newly diagnosed diabetic
patient might include these items:

• Urine sugar and acetone are
within normal limits

• Follow-up care has been
established

• The patient and his family have
been taught administration of
insulin or oral hypoglycemic,
urine testing, diet planning, and
skin care.

The criteria are printed on
8½"x11" salmon-colored cards
placed in the chart on top of the
nurses' record. Using card-weight
stock makes the sheet more
durable, and the color and
location make them easy to find.

As you already know, outcome criteria focus on the patient
and how he should be at discharge. Keeping this in mind, look
at what's written in the first column *above the heavy horizontal line.*

In this column, you see the specific outcome criteria or
elements for patients who've undergone appendectomies. All
of these elements pertain to that surgical procedure and are
written in measurable terms — under the categories health,
activity level, and knowledge.

Now let's look at the second column. The checkmarks in
this column indicate if compliance to specific criteria is expected all of the time or none of the time. As you can see,
compliance to the criteria listed for appendectomies is expected all of the time.

Occasional conditions make compliance impossible. These
exceptions — if there are any — are listed in the third column.

Column 4 contains instructions for the medical data analyst
or the person retrieving the necessary data. This column tells
— in very specific terms — what must be documented, and
where on the records it should be found.

*Remember, your documentation is the only proof you have
that a patient was cared for properly.* When the required data
doesn't appear on the patient's medical record, the audit
committee must assume that some deficiency in care exists.

What about complications?
Below the heavy horizontal line, almost everything about the
worksheet changes. To help you understand this, let's look at
the columns separately:

• *Column 1:* Instead of seeing criteria listed here, you now
see the complications that might occur in a patient after an
appendectomy.

• *Column 2:* This column indicates that complications are
never expected for any case, since one of your biggest responsibilities as a nurse is to prevent them.

• *Column 3:* Instead of listing exceptions as it did before,
Column 3 now shows you exactly what you're supposed to do
to prevent complications — or if they *do* occur, how to deal
with them and who to report them to.

• *Column 4:* This column gives instructions to the medical
data analyst. In very specific terms, it tells her what information relating to the complications must be documented and

where it should be located on the patient's records.

When the audit shows deficiency
Now you have an explanation of how the outcome criteria worksheet is set up. As I said earlier, the audit committee uses this sheet in evaluating patient care.

However, suppose a sampling of patient charts on the same topic shows that a large number of criteria are not being met — or that too many complications are occurring. The committee immediately looks for a reason. To pinpoint that reason — or the cause of the deficiency — they sometimes do a process audit, which focuses directly on the nursing care. (In some hospitals, process audits are done routinely, not just when problems arise.)

Examining the process criteria worksheet
As you can see on page 163, the process criteria worksheet is set up in much the same way as the outcome criteria worksheet. However, the *audit topic* on a process criteria worksheet usually specifies a problem, although it can specify a disease or surgical procedure if the audit's done routinely.

In our example of a routine process audit, the audit topic listed at the top of the worksheet is "lower abdominal surgery." The elements in the first column list the specific assessment and management criteria that you must meet in caring for a patient with lower abdominal surgery.

The second column lists how many times you're expected to comply with those criteria; the third column lists exceptions; and the fourth column lists instructions for the medical data analyst. (Of course, when your process audit is for a specific problem, the criteria relate only to that.)

What happens next?
By using the process criteria to evaluate your nursing care, the audit committee can better determine where the deficiency exists. They may then identify the problem and suggest ways that it can be corrected. Later on, of course, a reaudit, or follow-up study, is done to see if the problem has been solved.

Good documentation reveals good care
You now know something about audit committees and the criteria they establish to evaluate patient care. Keep this in

mind, however: The only way any committee can truly assess your patient's care is through accurate documentation.

If your documentation is poor, an audit of your patient's records may show deficiencies *where there were really none*. Don't let this happen. Apply what you've learned about documentation in this book. Then you'll never present anything but a clear — and accurate — picture of how you cared for your patients.

Remember these important rules about nursing audits:

1. **A nursing audit is not done to "put you under a magnifying glass." On the contrary, you should welcome an audit because it benefits you, the patient, other health-team professionals, and the hospital.**
2. **A properly done audit provides a way to improve patient care.**
3. **A properly done audit demonstrates deficiencies in hospital policies and procedures.**
4. **A properly done audit encourages coordination in planning between health-team members.**
5. **A properly done audit improves communication between departments.**
6. **A properly done audit encourages better documentation by explaining exactly what's expected.**
7. **A properly done audit provides direction for inservice educational programs.**
8. **A properly done audit points out where additional facilities, equipment, or staff are needed.**
9. **A properly done audit provides a way to study particular aspects of patient care.**
10. **Remember, the only way an audit committee can truly assess your patient's care is through your documentation. Make sure it gives them a clear and accurate picture of what you've done.**

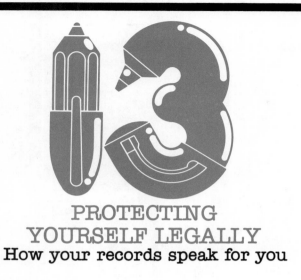

PROTECTING YOURSELF LEGALLY
How your records speak for you

BY AVICE KERR, RN, BA

YOU'RE A TRIAGE NURSE in the emergency department of a big city hospital. Early one evening, a middle-aged woman falls in the hospital parking lot and comes into the E.D. with a badly injured knee. You check her knee immediately, then ask her to wait to see a doctor.

Much to your surprise, the woman refuses to do so and leaves. What do you do? Should you enter it on your emergency department records?

Now, let's look at another case. This time you're a nurse in a busy medical/surgical unit. One morning, you answer a patient's call light and discover his roommate has fallen out of bed. How do you document this, after you've taken care of the emergency? Do you write *everything* that you think happened in the patient's progress notes? Or do you write only that you found the patient on the floor — and put the rest of the details about the incident in an incident report?

What you do or don't document in either of these cases could be important legally. So if you're at all uncertain, you need to read this chapter. In it, I'll tell you what to do in the cases above, as well as many others. I'll also explain how records can be used in a lawsuit — and how to protect yourself

Just in case

If, despite your best efforts, you do ever find yourself in court, remember that juries tend to believe nurses. Tell the truth, and have records to substantiate your statements.

The attorney will probably treat you with great courtesy, but don't get the idea he's trying to be fair. He's there to *win*. If he can, he will get you to say what he wants you to say. Be sure that you listen carefully to each question and fully understand it before you answer.

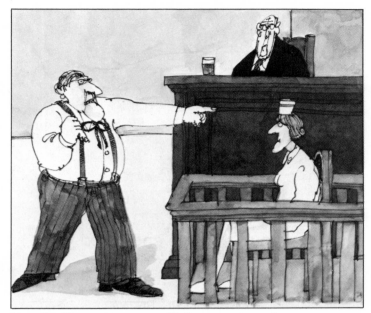

from liability, without sacrificing your integrity.

As an added bonus, this chapter will also include a special section about you and the law. It lists 15 of the most common questions posed to lawyers by nurses — and provides the answers.

That's where the goodies are

"Nurses' notes. That's where the goodies are!" I've heard this expression repeatedly from trial lawyers who handle body injury and medical malpractice cases. These lawyers, of course, are seeking evidence to support their clients' claims for damages.

Why do you suppose they look to nurses' notes for really convincing evidence? Here are several good reasons: When orders are written, the nurses' notes hold the only clue as to whether the orders were carried out and what the results were. Sometimes they are the *only* notes written with both the time and date on them. And they almost always offer the most detailed information on the patient.

How records are used legally

Before you write another note, consider the ways medical

records are used legally:
- to determine extent of injury in accident claims
- to show a series of events leading up to a patient's injury in the hospital, and determine who is to blame
- to show failure on the staff's part to use information available on the patient's record, and prove that the patient suffered as a result
- to show failure to transfer important information from one hospital department to another; for example, information showing that the patient is allergic to a particular drug or diagnostic dye
- to show failure to write clear medical orders.

Does all this frighten you? It shouldn't, if you're giving your patients quality care and documenting it properly. But so far in this book, you've learned only how your documentation — or lack of it — affects the *care* of your patients. What I want to teach you now is how it affects everyone involved *legally*.

Protect yourself and the hospital

Before I discuss how you can protect yourself in case of an unwarranted lawsuit, read the 15 legal questions nurses usually ask lawyers (pages 170 and 171).

Now do you have a better idea of where you stand legally? Then let's discuss some ways you can further protect yourself with good documentation.

Avoid basket terms

First, avoid using basket terms when you document. Be specific. For example, don't write that a patient is in "good condition." That could mean almost anything: that he's in no immediate danger, that he's getting better, or that he's ready for discharge.

What's more, if you're used to caring for very ill patients, your evaluation may differ decidedly from that of a nurse who's used to caring for patients who are not particularly ill. So, when you document an evaluation of your patient's condition, always include the specific findings that back up your evaluation: for example, write something like "ambulating in room without assistance."

Don't write that the patient had "a good night." Does this mean that he was comfortable and slept well? Or does it mean that he was quiet and didn't bother you? "A good night," "a

ANSWERS TO THE 15 LEGAL QUESTIONS NURSES USUALLY ASK

BY LORNE ELKIN ROZOVSKY, BA, LLB
Legal counsel, Nova Scotia Department of Health and
Member of the Faculty of Medicine,
Dalhousie University, Halifax, Canada

I ALWAYS INCLUDE a question-and-answer period during the seminars I give on nursing and the law, and the questions are almost always the same.

Here are the 15 most common questions — along with my answers.

TAKING ORDERS

Years ago, few nurses would have dared to say no to a doctor's order. Today, most of the nurses I talk to would not only dare to say no, they're looking for legal guidelines on how to go about it.

Can I legally refuse a doctor's order?

As a general rule, a nurse may not substitute her judgment for the doctor's. So the general answer to the question is no.

That does not mean you should blindly follow orders — particularly if you know something about the patient's condition that the doctor doesn't know.

Suppose, for example, that the doctor orders penicillin for a patient who, you know, is allergic to penicillin. In a case like this, the law expects you to inform the doctor before you carry out the order. In fact, if you don't inform the doctor, and the patient is injured as a result of the action ordered, *you could be considered negligent.*

But if the doctor confirms the order — despite your information — you must weigh your feelings. If it's a question of *judgment* (you simply disagree with the doctor's judgment), you'd better carry out the order anyway because the law doesn't permit you to substitute your nursing judgment for the doctor's medical judgment. Of course, you'll record the fact that you questioned the order and that the doctor confirmed it before you carried it out.

But if you feel that *no reasonable, prudent nurse would ever carry out the order,* you must refuse to carry it out. Naturally, you don't simply ignore the order. You record your decision and ask your supervisor for direction.

The doctors at our hospital keep delegating more and more to the nurses. How much can we legally do?

State and provincial laws and nurse practice acts have generally been unable to keep pace with the extended role of nurses. So it's hard to find specific guidelines.

Your best test in deciding whether to accept a delegated job is the same test the courts use: the test of reasonableness.

Let's say a doctor delegates a task; the nurse performs it; and the patient claims he was harmed by it.

The court will ask two questions:

• *Was the doctor acting reasonably* when he delegated the task? For its answer, the court will try to determine what other doctors would do in similar circumstances.

If other doctors wouldn't have delegated the task, the doctor in question may be considered negligent.

• *Was the nurse acting reasonably* when she accepted the task? The key to this answer is the education and experience of the nurse. If the nurse wasn't trained to do the task, she should have informed the doctor and refused the task. If she accepted the task without informing him of her lack of training, she alone could be considered negligent. If she told him but still accepted the task, they both could be considered negligent.

Should nurses accept medical orders over the telephone?

As a general rule, no. The danger of errors, patient injury, and lawsuits is obvious. And in a lawsuit that centers on the accuracy of a telephone order, either the doctor or the nurse will be held responsible, depending on which one the court feels has the better memory. Even a record of the telephone order may be questioned.

For a more specific answer, find out whether your hospital has bylaws, regulations, or policies dealing with this situation. Also find out whether your state or province has specific laws on telephone orders (a few do). *Failure to follow the law or hospital rules could be considered evidence of negligence* if a patient is injured because of confusion over a telephone order.

If your hospital doesn't have any policies regarding telephone orders, I'd advise you to request them. Even emergency orders should follow established procedure, to ensure that the order is understood and to require that the doctor confirm the order in writing as soon as possible.

THE CONSENTING PATIENT
Most nurses know that patients should understand and agree to any treatment before it's performed on them, but many nurses don't quite know what their role is in guaranteeing this patient right.

What is a nurse's responsibility for getting consent for treatment?
Except in an emergency in which the patient is unable to consent, every treatment requires the patient's consent.

For most nursing procedures, the nurse's responsibility is to explain the procedure. If the patient permits her to perform the procedure after she explains it, consent is implied. If the patient objects to the procedure, the nurse should accept that decision and inform the patient's doctor.

For many medical and surgical procedures, the patient must give explicit consent, and this is the kind of consent nurses usually ask me about.

In my answer, I always distinguish between *obtaining* consent and *witnessing* consent.

No nurse should ever take the responsibility for *obtaining* consent for a surgical procedure, because *obtaining* consent requires an explanation of the procedure and its risks. The nurse may not know exactly what procedure the surgeon is going to do. She may not know the risks that particular patient faces, or the risks of alternative procedures. If she takes the responsibility anyway and somehow misleads the patient about the nature of the procedure and its risks, she may

be included in a subsequent lawsuit.

Nurses may safely accept the responsibility for *witnessing* consent, however, because the witness to a consent has no legal liability in a subsequent lawsuit. Of course, the court may ask a nurse-witness to identify the patient's signature and to describe the patient's condition at the time he signed.

A legal gray area appears when nurses are asked to ensure that consent is properly obtained; that is, that consent is voluntary and that the patient is informed and able to give consent. If you're asked to do this, be sure that your hospital has an established procedure and then follow it carefully. Also, be sure you keep a record of your conversation with the patient, the questions you asked, the patient's response, and his condition at the time.

Can a sedated patient give consent?
This would be a dangerous assumption to proceed on. The danger is that the patient may not be capable of understanding the nature and risks of the procedure (or of not undergoing the procedure), in which case, his consent would not be valid.

What if a patient consents to one procedure then, during surgery, the surgeon considers another procedure necessary? Can the surgeon go ahead and do it?
If an emergency arises during the operation, the surgeon can (and should) perform all procedures necessary to meet the emergency.

Ordinarily, however, the surgeon can only perform the procedures consented to.

The problem is to devise a consent form that allows sufficient flexibility for the surgeon without being so broad it's meaningless.

KEEPING RECORDS
Nurses' notes are more than a current status report to help the health-care team plan its care. They are also an important legal record. Good notes can protect the

nurse and the hospital in the event of an unwarranted lawsuit.

What should nurses note, and how should this information be recorded?

What you should note is *all the information necessary to communicate the progress of the patient.* Your legal purpose is to document the fact that the patient's care met legally required standards. Good notes can thus refute a patient's unwarranted claim of negligence or malpractice.

How you should record this information *depends on your institution's system of charting.* As a minimum, the system should require:

• Notes made at the time of (or immediately after) the event recorded, with the time and date included.

• Notes written and signed by the person doing or seeing the event that's being recorded.

• Notes made in chronological order.

• Uniform abbreviations, understood by all members of the health-care team.

• Notes that are clear, concise, unambiguous, and accurate.

• Notes that are legible.

Do patients have a legal right to see their records?

Patients have this *right* in only two situations: First, in states and provinces that specifically give patients this right; second, in a legal case in which the court orders the hospital to divulge the record.

Of course, patients in any state or province *may* see their records with their doctors' or hospitals' permission.

Rather than focus on this question of legal rights, I think you should consider a more important issue, however. Usually, patients want to see their records only after they've begun to distrust the doctor or hospi-

tal staff for some reason. So, hospital staffs should work to restore their patients' trust and thus avoid more serious legal consequences.

ON THE WITNESS STAND

Understandably, most nurses don't want to go to court for *any* reason. So questions on this subject relate to the nurse's role both as a witness and as a defendant.

If called as a witness, do I have to divulge confidential information?

Generally, yes. In most states and in all Canadian provinces, the court can require a nurse to divulge confidential information.

If you are called as a witness, be sure to consult a lawyer about the law in your state before you take the witness stand.

And, on the stand, if you're asked about confidential information, inform the judge that the information was given to you within a confidential, professional relationship, and ask the judge for specific directions.

If I make a mistake while I'm following orders, isn't the hospital responsible?

The hospital may be legally responsible *along with you,* but this *doesn't* relieve you of responsibility.

When a nurse makes a mistake that injures a patient, both the hospital and the nurse can be sued for the damage she caused. And, if the hospital is forced to pay, *it can turn around and sue the nurse.* Clearly, a nurse must take responsibility for her own actions.

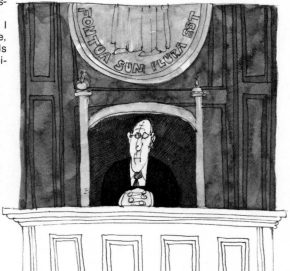

Do you mean I can be sued for any mistake I make?

No. The law doesn't expect you to be perfect — or even the best nurse in the world.

The law *does* expect you to give *reasonable* care: This is the duty you owe your patients.

Since the law doesn't expect perfection, a mistake or an error in judgment isn't necessarily negligence, even if patient injury results. A mistake *is* negligent if patient injury results *and if the court considers the mistake a failure to act like a reasonably prudent nurse* in the circumstances.

I'm a nursing instructor. If one of my students is negligent, am I responsible?

Ordinarily, no. You *would* be responsible if the court considered you negligent in supervising the student or in assigning a task you knew (or should have known) the student wasn't capable of doing. This means you should know every student's individual capabilities and not assume every student is capable of every task you've covered in class.

Am I responsible for other health-team members' negligence?

Again, you wouldn't ordinarily be responsible. However, on rare occasions you could be — for example, if you knew another team member was drunk and that his or her actions were likely to injure a patient. In this case, you would have a duty to the patient to take reasonable action to prevent his injury. If you failed to take action and the patient was thereby injured, you could be held responsible.

Let me emphasize, however, that this is rare. Ordinarily, you're entitled to rely on doctors, other nurses, and technicians to perform their duties in a reasonable and prudent manner, according to the standards of their own disciplines.

What about responsibility outside my job? Should I be afraid to be a Good Samaritan?

No. I don't know of any court decisions in the United States, Canada, or the United Kingdom that even deal with a volunteer nurse's actions at the scene of an accident.

Remember, a Good Samaritan nurse is only required to live up to reasonable and prudent nursing standards *in the circumstances*. The usual professional standards — under sterile conditions and with proper technical, pharmaceutical, and personnel support — would not be used as criteria.

A SIMPLE RULE

Is there any way I can minimize my chances of being sued?

Yes. Studies show that most malpractice suits contain two ingredients: The first is patient injury; the second is a breakdown in the doctor-patient, nurse-patient, or hospital-patient relationship.

What can you do? Obviously, you can work to prevent patient injury. Many injuries are preventable if the staff is educated to recognize potential causes of injury and how to prevent them. (The Maryland Hospital Association has designed a risk-management program that analyzes risks and then designs techniques for preventing them.)

Another thing you can do is to include patient education in your nursing care. Patients are less likely to sue if they have a realistic picture of the unavoidable risks they face.

Finally — and this is most important — you can work to prevent a breakdown in the nurse-patient relationship.

The simple rule to follow is to make a continuing effort *to treat the patients as human beings and not as cases.*

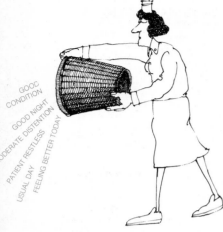

GOOD CONDITION
GOOD NIGHT
MODERATE DISTENTION
PATIENT RESTLESS
USUAL DAY
FEELING BETTER TODAY

Dumping basket terms
How do you recognize a "basket
term?" By the way it announces a
verdict without stating the
evidence. Evaluations are based
on specific information; by
presenting that information when
you document, you let the facts
speak for themselves.

good day," "a usual day": These terms are meaningful only
within a specific frame of reference. For example, suppose
you're caring for a patient who's in such severe pain that he
has trouble sleeping. For him, a "good night" may mean
nothing more than he got 2 hours of undisturbed sleep.

Never write that abdominal distention is "moderate" or
"marked." Instead, measure the circumference of the abdomen at the level of the umbilicus and record it. Then your notes
will show in measurable terms if the abdomen is increasing,
decreasing, or staying the same in size.

Don't write "patient feeling better today." How do you
know he's feeling better? If he simply moves a little easier or
smiles on more occasions, write that. Or if you decide he's
feeling better because he required less medication for pain,
write that. Remember, your notes take a "picture" of the
patient for the reader. Make them specific.

Avoid biased findings

Be careful that your documentation doesn't show bias. For
example, in a recent case, a patient was having petit mal
seizures several times each day. The nurses who documented
the seizures described them by saying "the patient stopped
what she was doing and stared into space."

Since the patient didn't seem to be responding to medication, a consultant was called in. He decided that she didn't
have epilepsy — or seizures — at all, and stopped all anticonvulsant medications.

Immediately the tone of the nurses charting changed. Instead of describing the patient's seizures as before, the notes
stated only that the patient's family said she had a seizure.
Every note afterward indicated that the nurses didn't really
believe the patient had a seizure. Anticonvulsant medications
were stopped, even though the patient and family still requested them.

Gradually over the next 24 hours, the episodes became more
severe until the patient had a grand mal seizure which would
not respond to medication. The final outcome was this: The
patient needed heavy medication and several hospitalizations
to bring her grand mal seizures under control.

We all tend to believe the "experts" and hate to think we are
out of step, but this is no excuse for allowing our observations
to be colored by someone else's opinion.

Make cautious but sensible judgments

In the past, when nurses were not supposed to have an opinion, we were all taught to write "appears" or "apparently" to avoid assuming the responsibility of making a forthright statement. I think that practice should be relegated to history.

We are taught to observe, so we should write what we observe without apology or subterfuge. For example, suppose you write that a patient's face was "apparently flushed." In court, a lawyer could make a great deal of the fact that you are "apparently" unsure whether your patient's face is flushed or not.

"Apparently asleep" is about the only "apparently" that makes sense to me. After all, if the patient is breathing like a sleeping person and has his eyes closed, you could presume that he is asleep. But there is really no way of knowing for sure unless you shake him awake and ask him if he was asleep.

Show continuity of care

Make sure your records show a continuous monitoring of your patient. For example, don't write down that you started an I.V. at 8 a.m., and never refer to that I.V. again until 4 p.m. What did you do about it between times? If nothing is charted, a patient could say that his I.V. site started to burn and swell 5 minutes after insertion and you did nothing about it.

For the patient who's not in need of constant care and continuous monitoring, such as one in a nursing home, you may have trouble charting meaningful notes. Flow sheets could show continuous monitoring of this type of patient. When you use them, always make sure you write the time, date, and your initials next to your entry.

Get a written policy

Make sure you have a *written* policy for everything you do, particularly if it may be considered controversial. For example, what are you expected to do if any of these situations arise:
- you're unable to reach the doctor when needed
- you're given orders for fluids or medications that are inappropriate for the patient
- a doctor gives you a verbal no-code order on a terminally ill patient
- you have a patient who refuses needed medication or

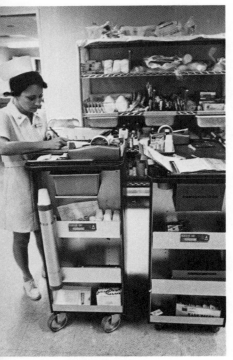

Medication tip
Do you remember the "Five Rights" for giving medication?
- right person
- right drug
- right dose
- right route
- right time

Here's another "right" to add to your list: *right reaction.*

If your patient might have an adverse reaction to a drug, be sure to check his condition frequently and to *chart your observations.* By doing this, you not only protect your patient, but you have a legal record that you've done so.

treatment, or leaves the hospital against medical advice
- you have standing orders for a medication or procedure that you no longer feel is warranted.

Remember when you follow the hospital's written policy for one of these situations, *always document that you followed it and what happened* in the proper time sequence.

For example, suppose you were unable to reach the doctor when needed urgently. Listing the time before every entry, you'd document:
- that you tried to contact the doctor but were unable to reach him.
- who took the message in the doctor's office.
- what doctor you contacted instead, and/or what other action you took.
- what happened as a result of all this and what you did about it.

Nursing tip: Any time you leave a message with someone in the doctor's office, note the time and the name of the person who took the message. If the message is urgent, your notes should state that this was explained to the person who took the message.

Now let's go back to the patient at the very beginning of this chapter — the middle-aged woman who left the emergency department without treatment.

What's the correct procedure to follow when you have a case like hers? Here's what I recommend:
- Make up a chart immediately, listing all the information the patient has given you about herself.
- Document any observations you made while she was with you, as well as what you did about them.
- Document that you notified the doctor, and asked the woman to wait.
- Get a written release signed by the patient, if possible.
- Document when she left and the reason she gave for leaving, if any.

Every line counts
The *order* in which you write your notes can be as important as *what* you write. For example, suppose your records are structured to show a chronological time sequence. What do you do when your note is out of order?

Don't ever ask a nurse to "save you a couple of lines," and

don't save empty lines for anyone else. Just write your note out of sequence and mark "late note" above it next to the time.

I can give you a good reason for this. In a malpractice suit, nothing pleases a plaintiff's lawyer more than finding a chart with vital information squeezed between the lines. He will have no trouble convincing a jury that, if the note was legitimate, it would've been charted chronologically in the first place.

Another important rule to remember to protect yourself is this: Never change your observation on a record to cover up for another professional's mistake. Chart the observations *only as you know them* — not what others tell you to write.

What to do about special forms

In the special section on legal questions and answers in this chapter, you learned what your responsibilities are obtaining and witnessing a patient's consent. But two other forms need your attention before I close this chapter. They are the patient instruction sheet, which I discussed in Chapter 11, and the incident report.

Charting the incident

Let's talk here about the incident report, which — as you know — enables you to give a full accounting of an incident that occurred in the hospital or on hospital property. (This report goes to the hospital administration.)

So I can better illustrate how to deal with this form, think back to the beginning of this chapter and the patient who was injured when he fell out of bed. After you take care of his injuries, how do you document the details of the accident — on the progress notes or on an incident report? Now I know that some hospital lawyers advise nurses not to write in the progress notes. In fact, they may even say that you shouldn't chart that you filled out an incident report.

Don't be misled into thinking you must protect only the hospital and not yourself and the patient. Anytime you're responsible for documenting an accident or medication error, write exactly what happened and what was done about it on both the progress notes and the incident report. Remember, most juries can understand human error; what they won't tolerate is an attempt to cover it up.

Never think that if you do not chart an incident or error,

A teaching tip
When instructing your patient in health care, how can you be sure he understands what you've told him? Suppose you're teaching a patient who's ready for discharge how to care for his leg wound. As you demonstrate the proper way to change his dressing, he nods and smiles brightly. When you ask him "Do you think you can do this without help?" he answers "Yes."

Now you can assume he's understood what you've shown him? No. Remember, some patients are too embarrassed to admit that they haven't understood. Others may not realize the instructions are something *they* should remember; instead, they think you're just telling them what *you* do. To get a clear picture of your patient's understanding, ask him to give a return demonstration in cases like this. Document that you've taught the patient what he needs to know only *after* he's shown that he can change his dressing unassisted.

there's no case. In law, you'll find a principle called "res ipsa loquitur" which is Latin for "the thing speaks for itself." In other words, it makes no difference if records say nothing about a patient falling out of bed. If he has bruises that are seen by family, friends, and roommates, he has a demonstrable injury on which a lawyer can build a case.

Some last words

I know I've given you a lot to consider in this chapter, but I don't want you to think only of lawsuits when you document patient care. Document to communicate the information health-team members need to give your patients the best possible care. If you do this, the record will automatically become the best defense against legal action. It'll show that you knew the patient's problems, that you implemented his care plan, and that you were alert for possible complications.

Remember these rules about protecting yourself legally:
 1. **Avoid using basket terms when you document. Be specific.**
 2. **Indicate in the record that you not only know what complications may occur but that you are seeking to prevent them.**
 3. **Document that you're taking safeguards to protect your patient; for example, putting side rails up and using safety belts where appropriate.**
 4. **Never let long periods of time go by without any charting. It may look like the patient was neglected during that time.**
 5. **Never insert notes between lines or leave an empty space for someone else to insert a note.**
 6. **If something goes wrong, first help the patient and report it to the doctor. Then document the mistake or accident in your progress notes and on the incident report.**
 7. **Always sign your name on any entry you've made on flow sheets or progress notes.**
 8. **Have a written policy for everything you do, especially if it may be considered controversial.**
 9. **Never change your documentation to cover up for someone else's mistakes.**
10. **Don't think only of possible lawsuits when you document; think instead of communicating needed information for quality patient care.**

SKILLCHECK 5

1. Your patient's surgical dressings are saturated with blood. He is pale, diaphoretic, and experiencing postural hypotension and tachycardia. Which documentation best meets legal requirements?
a) Patient is apparently shocky due to hypovolemia; vital signs unstable, skin appears cold and clammy.
b) Patient has lost a large amount of blood from his surgical site; vital signs deteriorating rapidly; condition seems critical.
c) Bright red bleeding from patient's surgical wound has saturated six abdominal dressings within 5 minutes. Skin is pale, diaphoretic; patient shows evidence of postural hypotension and tachycardia (see flow sheets).
d) Patient is experiencing hypovolemic shock due to arterial hemorrhage at surgical site. Vital signs indicate cardiac and renal failure imminent.

2. You're about to witness your patient signing a surgical consent, when he tells you he really didn't understand his doctor's explanation of his surgery. What do you do?
a) Notify the doctor that additional explanation is needed before witnessing the consent.
b) Explain the procedure, then witness the consent.
c) Tell your patient that additional explanation will be given, but consent is necessary now.
d) Document that you are unable to get a written consent at this time.

3. You receive a medication order for your patient which you feel greatly exceeds the safe dosage range. What do you do first?
a) Contact the doctor and discuss the situation.
b) Refuse to give the medication and document your refusal.
c) Give the medication and document that you followed medical orders.
d) Refuse to give the medication and document nothing.

4. Which of these charting situations is most likely to involve you in legal difficulties?
a) Having your patient sign a release form if he's leaving the hospital against medical advice.
b) Charting out of sequence and marking it a "late note."

c) Charting that your patient's condition is progressing normally.
d) Using flow sheets to document continuous monitoring of your patient.

5. You have completed your charting and notice you've made an error. What should you do?
a) Blacken the error out with ink.
b) Erase the error.
c) Leave the error and write in the correction.
d) Draw one line in ink through the error and make the correction.

6. What documentation (if any) should you make if an accident occurs while you're giving patient care?
a) None, to protect yourself legally.
b) Chart the facts only as you know them on the incident report and progress notes.
c) Chart the accident facts only on the incident report.
d) Chart the accident facts only on the progress notes.

7. You're working in a coronary care unit and want to know what standards of nursing care your peers have decided on for a patient with an MI. Where do you look for this information?
a) Nursing audit outcome criteria
b) Nursing audit process criteria
c) Nursing audit structure criteria
d) Nursing audit complication criteria.

8. How can you, a staff nurse, best help an audit committee make an honest appraisal of your nursing care?
a) Be sure that your documentation is thorough and accurate.
b) Request that a committee member supervise your care for 1 day.
c) Explain how your charting deficiencies are not really care deficiencies.
d) Ask to serve as an audit committee member.

9. You're planning discharge care for your patient and want to be sure you know what his health, activity level, and knowledge should be when he leaves. Where can you look for guidance?
a) Nursing audit outcome criteria
b) Nursing audit process criteria
c) Nursing audit structure criteria
d) Nursing audit complication criteria.

(Answers on page 181)

ANSWERS TO SKILLCHECKS

ANSWERS TO SKILLCHECK 1 (page 33)

Situation 1
b) Collect enough significant data to make an accurate assessment.

Situation 2
c) Document information obtained from interview on the assessment sheet. Also include identified problems and nursing orders on the care plan to ensure consistent care.

Situation 3
d) After considering several approaches, select and indicate the one approach to be used.

Situation 4
c) When documentation indicates the approaches are not solving the problem, revise the approaches on the care plan.

Situation 5
a) Source-oriented records are frequently kept according to sequence rather than according to problem; they always contain separate notes from each professional group.

Situation 6
c) Both source-oriented and problem-oriented medical records should contain initial assessment information.

Situation 7
d) A combination of source- and problem-oriented systems contains problem oriented essentials, but includes separate sections for one or more professional groups.

Situation 8
a) When a nurse writes source-oriented records, she doesn't always separate the patients' problems by paragraph. Instead, she may group them altogether, as shown in our question.

ANSWERS TO SKILLCHECK 2 (page 75)

Situation 1
d) Convey a feeling of personal concern. Strive to improve the patient's internal environment for a more effective interview.

Situation 2
a) Questions that stimulate explanations are more effective than questions easily answered by "yes" or "no." Avoid leading questions.

Situation 3
d) Gain control over the environment so both you and your patient will give full attention to the interview.

Situation 4
d) Never encourage a patient to reveal more about herself than she's comfortable revealing.

Situation 5
c) When you've come to the end of your interview, share what you feel the interview has accomplished, what you and he consider to be his needs, and what both of you plan to do about them.

Situation 6
c) It's important to record your patient's usual patterns of daily living so you can plan her care around them.

Situation 7
a) Never jump to a conclusion when you make an observation. Obtain sufficient information to make an effective decision.

Situation 8
d) Record the reason for hospitalization as the patient sees it. You may even want to use the same words.

Situation 9
d) Be thorough when you document physical assessment findings. Remember, do not use vague terms.

ANSWERS TO SKILLCHECK 3 (page 113)

Situation 1
b) Problems #2, 4, and 5 have been resolved. Problems #1 (peptic ulcer) and #3 (diabetes) are active.

Situation 2
d) The approach is not specific for time and the need for a return demonstration.

Situation 3
b) Insufficient data base is the first problem identified. It should be written on the problem list and/or care plan to allow quick resolution.

Situation 4

a) You can identify a symptom as an active problem when the doctor has not yet confirmed the medical diagnosis.

Situation 5

c) If you can't get the information you need during the interview, check out the nonverbal messages you convey to your patient to see if they're negative.

ANSWERS TO SKILLCHECK 4 (page 155)

Situation 1

d) *O* data gives objective information — that which you've collected when you've observed or inspected your patient.

Situation 2

b) *E* data gives evaluative information. Here's where you document your patient's response to your intervention, either positive or negative.

Situation 3

b) *A* data indicates the conclusions you've come to about *S* and *O* data. You may even say you don't know what's going on, because sometimes you're not sure.

Situation 4

c) Always write your notes in *specific* descriptive terms which cannot be confused or misinterpreted.

Situation 5

b) Unless you're instructed otherwise, write on your patient's progress notes whenever you've observed a change in his condition.

Situation 6

a) In the source-oriented system, always write separate narrative paragraphs about each problem that you may be documenting.

Situation 7

b) Pull out all the information your patient needs to know from your discharge summary and write the instructions in a way she will understand.

Situation 8

c) To write a POMR discharge summary, you'll make all your entries in the SOAPIER style. Each of the patient's problems will be discussed.

ANSWERS TO SKILLCHECK 5 (page 179)

Situation 1

c) Don't use "basket terms" when you document. Always include the specific findings that indicate the patient's condition.

Situation 2

a) Don't witness this consent since the patient is not well-informed. First notify the doctor, who has legal responsibility for explaining surgical procedures.

Situation 3

a) You shouldn't blindly follow orders. If you feel that no reasonable, prudent nurse would carry out the order, you should *first* inform the doctor, who then may change the order.

Situation 4

c) Don't use vague terms when charting. "Progressing normally" may be interpreted in many ways.

Situation 5

d) Legally, an error on a chart should be corrected by drawing one line in ink through the error and making the correction.

Situation 6

b) Any time you're responsible for documenting an accident, write exactly what you know happened and what was done about it on both the progress notes and an incident report. Never think if you do not chart an accident there's no case.

Situation 7

b) Process criteria focus on nursing care. In this case, they outline exactly what standards you follow when caring for any patient with an MI.

Situation 8

a) By calculating what percentage of patient records meets the standards, the audit committee can determine the quality of care. This is true only if the retrievable data reflects an accurate picture.

Situation 9

a) Outcome criteria focus on the patient and the end result of his care. They indicate how the patient should be at discharge in terms of his health, activity level, and knowledge.

NURSING DATA BASE
(Assessment)

SECTION I: Date _12/16/77_   Time _2 PM_   Name _Mary Anthony_

Mode _litter from doctor's office_   Age _45_

T _99⁸_ P _88_ R _18_ BP _120/80_ Ht _66"_ Wt _115 lbs._

Diet _1800 cal ADA_ Bloodwork: Yes _X_ No _____ Urinalysis: Yes _X_ No _____

Prosthesis: Glasses _—_ Contact lenses _Yes_ Dentures _No_ Other _none_

General orientation to hospital environment by: _B. Frick R.N_   _12/16/77_
                                                Signature   Date

Section I must be completed and signed by an RN or LPN on all admissions.

SECTION II: Date _12/16/77_   Time _2³⁰ PM_

Reason for hospitalization or chief complaint: _Severe RLQ abdominal pain_
Vomited x 1

Duration of this problem/onset: _Dull pain → 10 hrs Severe pain → last 3 hrs._

Admitting diagnosis: _Appendicitis_

Previous hospitalizations and illnesses:

Date	MD	Where	Type of illness or surgery and reaction
1975	E. Jones	Western Mem.	Diagnosis of Diabetes — no problems
1976	R. Schroder	Somerset Paril.	Treatment of retinal hemorrhages c̄ Laser — no problems

Family Health History:

Diabetes _F↓_ Heart _m ↑_ Cancer _aunt ↓_ Kidney _neg_ T.B. _neg_ COPD _neg_

Asthma _neg_ Epilepsy _neg_ Psychiatric _neg_ Other _none_

Social history of alcohol _none_ Smoking _does not smoke_

Allergies (what and type of reaction) _dog hair — congestion_

Medications code: A — Sent home with family; B — May be self-administered; C — Not brought in with patient.

Name	Code	Dose and time	Time of last dose	Patient's understanding of purpose
Orinase	C	0.25 g. bid	7PM 12/15/77	Used in conjunction c̄ ADA diet to control DM

Review of Systems:

EENT _PEERLA, ENT — no discharge or signs of infection, no gland enlargement_

Neurological _reflexes normal, patient denies any history of numbness or tingling_

Pulmonary _no rales or wheezes; denies cough or congestion_

Cardiovascular _HR-88, NSR. No murmurs noted. Denies history of cardiac disease_

GI _Severe RLQ pain for 3 hrs. Psoas sign positive. Rebound tenderness_
noted. Constipation this past week.
GU _No nocturia. Denies frequency or urgency_

Skin _Dry. No bruises, scabs or ulcerations_

Mental/emotional status _calm, despite severe pain_
Reproductive _LMP 12/5/77 Periods decreasing in amt. over past year_
Signature for minimal assessment _B. Frick RN_
Section II must be completed and signed by an RN (both Sections I and II must be completed on short-term admissions).

SECTION III: Date _12/16/77_   Time _2³⁰ PM_
Patterns:
    Hygiene _Bathes early PM before work._
    Rest/sleep _Sleeps 6-8 hrs. Thur — Sun retires at 3ᴬᴹ. Mon - Wed. — 11ᴾᴹ_
    Activity status _No ambulation problems_
    Elimination habits _Bowel = occ. constipation Bladder = no problems._
    Meals/diet _1800 cal ADA - occ. use of diabetic sweets_
    Health practices _Yearly PAP smear. Monthly SBE See family doctor for DM_
    Typical daily profile: _Lives alone. Sleeps till 10ᴬᴹ Breakfast @ 12ᴺᴼᴼᴺ. Dancing_
    twice a week. Yoga on Thursday. Main meal at 4ᴾᴹ. Light snack
    7-8 PM before show. Orinase at 1130ᴬᴹ & 7 PM
Information obtained from: Patient _X_ Family _____ Previous records _____
COMMENTS: _Patient concerned about cause of abdominal pain_
The possibility of surgery has been discussed and she
verbalizes a good understanding of the implications

Signature _B. Frick R.N._
Section III — Completed by an RN. (Sections I, II and III must be completed on all patients except those defined by policy as
short-term.)

NAME _Mary Anthony_

AGE ____45____

PATIENT PROBLEM LIST

DATE ONSET	NO.	PAST, CHRONIC, OR ACTIVE PROBLEMS	INITIAL	DATE RESOLVED	INACTIVE OR RESOLVED PROBLEMS
12/16/77	1	Appendicitis ——12/16/77——7 Appendectomy	BF RN		
Child hood	2	Allergy to dog hair	BF RN		
1975	3	Diabetes mellitus	BF RN		
	4	————————————————7	BF RN.	1976	Retinal hemor- rhages 2% #3

PATIENT CARE PLAN

DATE STARTED	D/C'd	PROBLEM	DIRECTIVES
12/16/77	12/16/77	No 1 Appendicitis	A) Measure vital signs Q 2 h
			B) Semi-Fowlers position
			Offer pain med Q 4 h
			Ice bag R L Q
			NPO to decrease peristalsis
			Partial bath . B R P
			C) Teach C.T. + D.B. + leg exercises once
			patient is comfortable after pain med.
			Explain R.R. procedure + shave prep.
			Told patient to use call light when
			needing assistance
			Pt. + family told by Dr. that surgery
			essential. Scheduled for O.R. at 5³⁰ ᴾᴹ
			Dr. told patient + family, that when
			diabetes is controlled, surgery is no
			greater risk than c̄ non-diabetic
			B. Frick R.N.
12/16/77		No 3 Diabetes mellitus	A) Urine reductions Q.I.D. AC + HS. Document
			on diabetic flow sheet
			✓ Lab reports of Blood sugar + electrolytes
			B) Monitor IV 5% dextrose in water
			Be alert for signs of hypoglycemic
			reaction, ie, sweating, trembling,
			headache, diplopia. Notify doctor.
			Be alert for signs of dehydration, ie
			dry warm skin, cracked lips, ↓ urine.
			Measure I + O Q 8 h
			C) Pt. told sub Q insulin will be given
			temporarily
			B. Frick R.N.

PATIENT CARE PLAN

NAME **Mary Anthony**

AGE **45**

DATE STARTED	D/C'd	PROBLEM	DIRECTIVES
12/16/77	12/17/77	No. 1 Appendectomy	A) Monitor vitals signs Q 1 hr x4 then q.i.d. B) Ambulate pt. in A.M. Cough, turn, deep breathe and leg exercises Q 2° til ambulatory. Offer pain med Q 4 h. Oral hygiene and ice chips when fully reacted. Dressing Q 2 h for hemorrhage. C) Instructed husband to request assistance from staff at any time.
12/16/77		No. 3 Diabetes mellitus	A) Continue on sub q insulin thru 12/17/77 back on Orinase 0.25 g b.i.d. 12/18/77 B) Pt. and husband informed of this C) Continue preop plan. *M. Reilly, R.N.*
12/17/77		NO. 1 APPENDECTOMY	A) MEDICATE WITH DEMEROL FOR PAIN. CHANGE DRESSING Q. DAY. CLEANSE INCISION WITH BETADINE, REDRESS WITH STERILE 4 X 4's. NO BINDER OBSERVE INCISION FOR SIGNS OF INFLAMMATION, I.E., PURULENT, FOUL SMELLING DRAINAGE, REDNESS TEACH PATIENT HOW TO CLEANSE WOUND AND REDRESS. SUPERVISE AND ✓ RETURN DEMONSTRATION. B) ENCOURAGE AMBULATION — NOT PROLONGED SITTING. C) INSTRUCT PATIENT IN ACTIVITIES PERMITTED FOLLOWING DISCHARGE, I.E., LIGHT HOUSE HOLD TASKS — DISHES, DUSTING. NOT PERMITTED TO WASH CLOTHES, SCRUB FLOORS OR RUN SWEEPER FOR 3 WEEKS. SEXUAL ACTIVITY RESTRICTED FOR 3 WEEKS. INSTRUCT TO SEE PHYSICIAN AT HIS OFFICE IN 3 WEEKS. *P. Nice, R.N.*
12/17/77		NO. 3 DIABETES MELLITUS	A) INITIATE REFERRAL TO DIABETIC NURSE SPECIALIST FOR KNOWLEDGE ASSESSMENT. *P. Nice, R.N.*

50 COMMONLY CONFUSED ABBREVIATIONS

Although abbreviations help save time and space, they can cause charting confusion if you use them improperly. Some common abbreviations may stand for several things, as you see in the list below. For example, when the patient chart reads *ARF*, does it mean *acute respiratory failure*, or *acute rheumatic fever*? Such ambiguities could lead to serious error,

with disastrous consequences for your patients.

How can you avoid problems with abbreviations? Be doubly careful when interpreting them. If you're in doubt, check with the doctor. When writing, don't make up your own abbreviations. Always stick to the conventional ones. Remember, on those portions of the chart most likely to be used for legal purposes, always write out the entire word.

Here are some abbreviations most likely to be confused:

AHD
arteriosclerotic heart disease
autoimmune hemolytic disease

ARF
acute respiratory failure
acute rheumatic fever

AS
aortic sounds
aortic stenosis
aqueous solution
aqueous suspension
arteriosclerosis
astigmatism

BS
blood sugar
bowel sounds
breath sounds

CA
calcium
cancer
cathode
caucasian adult
chronological age

CC
caucasian child
chief complaint
color and circulation
common cold
creatinine clearance
critical condition

CF
cardiac failure
cystic fibrosis

CHD
childhood disease
congenital heart disease
coronary heart disease

CI
cardiac insufficiency
cerebral infarction

CLD
chronic liver disease
chronic lung disease

CP
capillary pressure
cerebral palsy
certified prosthetist
child psychiatrist
chronic pyelonephritis
closing pressure (spinal tap)
constant pressure
cor pulmonale
creatinine phosphate

CT
circulation time
clotting time
coated tablet
compressed tablet
corneal transplant

DD
differential diagnosis
discharge by death
discharge diagnosis
dry dressing

DM
diabetes mellitus
diastolic murmur

DOA
date of admission
dead on arrival

ECF
extended care facility
extracellular fluid

EOM
external otitis media
extraocular movements

ER
emergency room
equivalent roentgen
expiratory reserve
external rotation

GC
general circulation
general condition
gonorrhea (gonococcus)

HS
heart sounds
herpes simplex
hour of sleep
house surgeon

IA
internal auditory
intra-arterial
intra-articular

ID
identification
ineffective dose
initial dose
inside diameter
intradermal

IM
infectious mononucleosis
internal medicine
intramedullary
intramuscularly

LE
left eye
Le prep (lab test)
lower extremity
lupus erythematosus

LOM
left otitis media
limitation of motion
loss of movement

LSB
left scapular border
left sternal border

MD
manic depression
medical doctor
muscular dystrophy
myocardial disease

MI
mental illness
mitral insufficiency
myocardial infarction
myocardial ischemia

MM
malignant melanoma
medial malleolus
mucous membrane
multiple myeloma
myeloid metaplasia

MS
mitral sounds
mitral stenosis
morphine sulfate
multiple sclerosis
musculoskeletal

NP
nasopharynx
nerve palsy
neuropsychiatry
new patient
not palpable

NR
nerve root
nonreactive
no report
no respiration
no resuscitation
normal range
normal reaction
not refillable
not remarkable

OD
every day
occupational disease
overdose
right eye

PA
pernicious anemia
primary amenorrhea
prolonged action
pulmonary artery

PAP
Papanicolaou's smear
passive aggressive personality
primary atypical pneumonia
pulmonary artery pressure

PE
pelvic exam
physical education
physical exam
point of entry
pulmonary embolism

PND
paroxysmal nocturnal dyspnea
post nasal drip

PO
by mouth
phone order
postop

PP
partial pressure
peripheral pulses
postpartum
postprandial
presenting problem

PR
perfusion rate
peripheral resistance
presbyopia
pressoreceptor
progress report
pulse rate

RA
renal artery
repeat action
rheumatoid arthritis
right arm
right atrium

RD
Raynaud's disease
respiratory disease
retinal detachment
right deltoid

RE
rear end (accident)
rectal examination
regional enteritis
right eye

RHD
relative hepatic dullness
rheumatic heart disease

ROM
range of motion
right otitis media

SD
septal defect
shoulder disarticulation
spontaneous delivery
standard deviation
sudden death

SH
self help
serum hepatitis
shoulder
sinus histiocytosis
social history

SOB
see order book
shortness of breath

SR
schizophrenic reaction
sedimentation rate
sinus rhythm
stretch reflex
system review

TM
temperature by mouth
tempromandibular
tender midline
transmetatarsal
tympanic membrane

A BRIEF GUIDE TO ASSESSMENT

No matter how assessment procedures may vary, all of them require a systematic approach. This sample chart, though by no means complete, shows how you might organize your own assessments by categories: *interviewing, observing,* and *inspecting.*

ASK ABOUT	OBSERVE (look, listen, smell)	INSPECT (touch)
Head		
visual disturbances	facial expressions (for example, grimace)	facial symmetry
headache	skin texture and color	edema
dizziness	eye position, sclera color	enlarged nodes
nosebleeds	breath odors	
hoarseness	discharge from ears, nose, or eyes	
ringing in ears	ulcerations	
pain (other than headache)		
Breast		
lumps or masses	symmetry	masses
pain	color	engorgement
	discharge or bleeding from nipples	
Lung		
chronic cough	chest symmetry	lung sounds
spitting up blood	lung sounds	(with stethoscope)
sputum	pursed-lip breathing	
pain	cough: type and frequency	
recent chest X-ray	sputum: amount, color, consistency	
	retraction, if any	
	respiratory rate and depth	
CV		
shortness of breath	dyspnea	all pulses
pain in calves or chest	arrhythmias	(bilaterally)
ankle swelling	diaphoresis	arrhythmias
	ankle edema	(with stethoscope)
	cyanosis	abdominal
	neck-vein distention	pulsations
		edema
GI		
change in bowel habits	emesis	bowel sounds
vomiting (amount and color)	distention	(with stethoscope)
bloody stools	any vasculature	masses
abdominal pain	jaundice	
	hernias	
	blood in stool	
GU		
frequency, urgency, hesitancy	amount and character of urine	bladder distention
blood in urine	hematuria, pyuria	swelling of
painful urination	discharge	external genitalia
Gyn		
pregnancies	discharge	
cramps	lesions	
menopause		
discharge		
lesions		
Extremities		
numbness	rashes	rashes
tingling,	color	ROM
difficulty walking,	(cyanosis, jaundice)	crepitus
any weakness	edema	edema
	lacerations	grip strength
	bruises	pulses
	ulcerations	
	pigmentation	
Neuropsychological		
depression	behavior (depressed, withdrawn, euphoric)	grip strength
insomnia	tone of voice	reflexes
anxiety	orientation (to time, place, and person)	(with reflex hammer)
	unusual body movements	
	posturing	
	verbal expressions (suicide threat)	

INDEX

Page numbers followed by the letter "t" indicate both tabular and marginal material.

BIBLIOGRAPHY

Berni, Rosemarian, and Helen Readey. *Problem-Oriented Medical Record Implementation.* St. Louis, C. V. Mosby Company, 1974.

Bjorn, J. C., and H. D. Cross. *The Problem-Oriented Private Practice of Medicine.* Chicago, Modern Hospital Press, 1970.

Bower, Fay Louise. *The Process of Planning Nursing Care*, 2nd ed. St. Louis, C. V. Mosby Company, 1977.

Fowkes, William C. Jr., and Virginia K. Hunn. *Clinical Assessment for the Nurse Practitioner.* St. Louis, C. V. Mosby Company, 1973.

Friedman, Harold, ed., and Solomon Papper, ed. *Problem-Oriented Medical Diagnosis.* Boston, Little, Brown and Company, 1975.

Froebe, Doris J., and R. Joyce Bain. *Quality Assurance Programs and Controls in Nursing.* St. Louis, C. V. Mosby Company, 1976.

Hurst, J. Willis, ed., and H. Kenneth Walker. *The Problem-Oriented System.* Baltimore, Williams & Wilkins Company, 1972.

Johnson, Mae M., and Mary L. Davis. *Problem-Solving in Nursing Practice.* Iowa, William C. Brown Company, 1975.

Kerr, Avice. *Medical Hieroglyphs: Abbreviations and Symbols.* California, Enterprise Publications, 1970.

Larkin, Patricia, and Barbara Backer. *Problem-Oriented Nursing Assessment.* New York, McGraw-Hill Book Company, 1976.

Little, Dolores E., and Doris L. Carnevalli. *Nursing Care Planning*, 2nd ed. Philadelphia, J. B. Lippincott Company, 1976.

Marram, Gwen D., and Margaret W. Schelgel. *Primary Nursing: A Model for Individualized Care.* St. Louis, C. V. Mosby Company, 1974.

Mayers, Marlene G., et. al. *Quality Assurance for Patient Care: Nursing Perspectives.* New York, Appleton-Century-Crofts, 1977.

Mitchell, Pamela. *Concepts Basic to Nursing.* New York, McGraw-Hill Company, 1973.

Neelon, Francis A., and George J. Ellis. *A Syllabus of Problem-Oriented Patient Care.* Boston, Little, Brown and Company, 1974.

Phaneuf, Maria C. *The Nursing Audit: Self-Regulation in Nursing Practice*, 2nd ed. New York, Appleton-Century-Crofts, 1976.

Readey, Helen, et. al. *Introduction to Nursing Essentials: A Handbook.* St. Louis, C. V. Mosby Company, 1977.

Vaughn-Wrobel, Beth C., and Betty Henderson. *The Problem-Oriented System in Nursing: A Workbook.* St. Louis, C. V. Mosby Company, 1976.

Vitale, Barbara A., et. al. *Problem Solving Approach to Nursing Care Plans: A Program.* St. Louis, C. V. Mosby Company, 1974.

Walker, H. Kenneth, ed., et. al. *Applying the Problem-Oriented System.* Baltimore, Williams & Wilkins, 1973.

Walter, Judith Bloom, ed., et. al. *Dynamics of Problem-Oriented Approaches: Patient Care and Documentation.* Philadelphia, J. B. Lippincott Company, 1976.

Weed, Lawrence L. *Medical Records, Medical Education, and Patient Care.* Chicago, Year Book Medical Publishers, 1970.

Woolley, F. Ross, et. al. *Problem-Oriented Nursing.* New York, Springer Publishing Company, 1974.

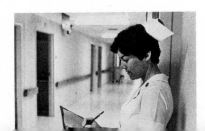